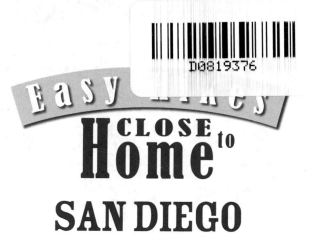

Easy Hikes

Home CLOSE to

SAN DIEGO

including
North, South, and East Counties

SHERI MCGREGOR

MENASHA RIDGE PRESS
Birmingham, Alabama

This book is meant only as a guide to select trails in the San Diego area and does not guarantee hiker safety in any way—you hike at your own risk. Neither Menasha Ridge Press nor Sheri McGregor is liable for property loss or damage, personal injury, or death that result in any way from accessing or hiking the trails described in the following pages. Please be aware that hikers have been injured in the San Diego area. Be especially cautious when walking on or near boulders, steep inclines, and drop-offs, and do not attempt to explore terrain that may be beyond your abilities. To help ensure an uneventful hike, please read carefully the introduction to this book, and perhaps get further safety information and guidance from other sources. Familiarize yourself thoroughly with the areas you intend to visit before venturing out. Ask questions, and prepare for the unforeseen. Familiarize yourself with current weather reports, maps of the area you intend to visit, and any relevant park regulations.

Copyright © 2009 Sheri McGregor
All rights reserved
Printed in the United States of America
Published by Menasha Ridge Press
Distributed by Publishers Group West
First edition, first printing

ISBN 978-0-89732-722-0

Cover by Scott McGrew
Cover photo by Sheri McGregor
Text design by Annie Long
Maps by Sheri McGregor, Scott McGrew, and Steve Jones
All interior photos by Sheri McGregor

Menasha Ridge Press
P.O. Box 43673
Birmingham, AL 35243
www.menasharidge.com

Contents

4 **AUTHOR'S NOTE**

5 **INTRODUCTION**

8 **TRAIL RECOMMENDATIONS**

13 **COAST**

14 **Hike 1:** Bayside Trail
15 **Hike 2:** La Jolla: Coast Walk Trail
21 **Hike 3:** La Jolla Shores: Tide Pools Walk
24 **Hike 4:** Torrey Pines State Reserve: Guy Fleming Trail
27 **Hike 5:** San Elijo Lagoon: La Orilla Trailhead to Rios Avenue Trail
31 **Hike 6:** Batiquitos Lagoon Trail

34 **MOUNTAINS**

35 **Hike 7:** Laguna Mountains: Sunset Trail
38 **Hike 8:** Inaja Memorial Trail
41 **Hike 9:** Santa Ysabel Open Space Preserve East:
      Kanaka Loop Trail
45 **Hike 10:** Palomar Mountain: Observatory Trail

49 **INLAND**

50 **Hike 11:** Lake Morena Trail
54 **Hike 12:** Miramar Reservoir Loop
57 **Hike 13:** Los Penasquitos Canyon Preserve:
      West End to Waterfall Loop
62 **Hike 14:** Del Dios Gorge Trail
65 **Hike 15:** Lake Poway Loop
69 **Hike 16:** Blue Sky Trail to Lake Ramona
74 **Hike 17:** Lake Hodges: North Shore Trail
77 **Hike 18:** Elfin Forest Recreational Reserve: Botanical Loop
80 **Hike 19:** Discovery Lake and Hills Loop
84 **Hike 20:** Lake Dixon: Shore View Trail
88 **Hike 21:** Los Jilgueros Preserve Trail
92 **Hike 22:** Wilderness Gardens Preserve: Combined Trails Loop

Author's Note

Sheri McGregor

These easy hikes from my published collection (plus new hikes) provide detailed opportunities for novice hikers to start enjoying the local outdoors. So many readers tell me they are tired of boring treadmills and high-priced gym memberships. Get outside where the hush of the breeze lulls you, the birds cheer you on, and beautiful views await.

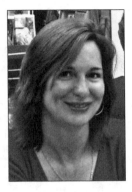

In nature, we experience sounds and images that capture our attention involuntarily and relax us. This makes the natural world a wonderful respite. The calm that comes from spending time in nature is also associated with improved memory, increased attention span, and positive benefits for people who are stressed. It has long been known that just viewing natural images and sounds decreases healing time.

I've hiked among the trees and observed wildlife and the changing seasons here in San Diego my whole life. Feeling my feet connect to Mother Earth with every step has always brought me joy. I hope that you, too, find the natural areas of these easy hikes will soothe your stress, allow you to clear your head, and get physically fit. Enjoy these easy San Diego trails with family and friends for peaceful bonding time. When you're ready for more advanced hikes, my books, *60 Hikes within 60 Miles: San Diego,* and *Day & Overnight Hikes: Anza Borrego Desert State Park,* will be there to guide you.

Please visit my Web site (**www.SanDiegoHikes.com**), and send me a note about your hiking experiences. I love to hear from readers and fellow hikers.

Introduction

Welcome to *Easy Hikes Close to Home: San Diego*. This title in the *Easy Hikes* series is organized according to three regions: Coast; Mountains; and Inland.

Numbered map icons on the inside front cover locate each primary trailhead and are keyed to the table of contents and narrative text for each trail. On the inside back cover, a map legend defines symbols for parking, restrooms, trail features, and other details. Armed with this handy guidebook, you can quickly head out the door and, well, take a hike!

OVERVIEW

Mileage shown for each hike corresponds to the total distance from start to finish, for loops, out-and-backs, figure eights, or a combination of shapes. You can shorten or extend some of them with connecting trails.

HIKING ESSENTIALS

Boots should be your footwear of choice. Sport sandals are popular, but they leave much of your foot exposed and vulnerable to hazardous plants, thorns, rocks, and sharp twigs.

When it comes to water, err on the side of excess. Hydrate prior to your hike, carry (and drink) six ounces of water for every mile you plan to hike, and hydrate after the hike. Pack along a couple of small bottles of water even for short hikes. You may decide to linger on the trail, or take an alternate route and extend your time outdoors.

Always plan for unpredictable scenarios by carrying these items, in addition to water:

Map

Compass

Basic first-aid supplies, such as Band-Aids and aspirin

Knife

Windproof matches or a lighter and fire starter

Snacks

Flashlight with extra batteries

Rain protection and a sweater or windbreaker, even in warm weather

Sun protection

Insect repellent

Whistle

GENERAL TIPS

The whole point of your outing is to enjoy nature, fresh air, and exercise. Here are a few tips to enhance your excursion:

- Avoid weekends and traditional holidays if possible; otherwise, go early in the morning. Trails that are packed in the summer are often clear during the colder months and during rainy times (but never hike during a thunderstorm).

- Before you hit the trail, double-check your map, and don't set out on the trail until you have the information you need.

- Once on the trail, be careful at overlooks, stay back from the edge of outcrops, and be absolutely sure of your footing wherever you are.

- Hike on open trails only. Respect trail and road closures, avoid trespassing on private land, and obtain permits if required. Leave gates as you found them or as marked.

- Stay on the existing trail, and avoid any littering.

- When hiking with children, use common sense to judge a child's capacity to hike a particular trail, and expect that the child may tire and need to be carried. Make sure children are adequately clothed for the weather, have proper shoes, and are protected from the sun with sunscreen. Kids dehydrate quickly, so make sure you have plenty of fluids for everyone.

- Take your time along the trails, whether you are doing one of this guide's short hikes or hours-long treks. In other words:

Don't miss the trees for the forest. You may finish some of the "hike times" long before or after that suggested in the Overview box. A short-distance hike with a lot of up-and-downs may take more time and energy than a longer, flatter hike.

- Participate in some online wildlife observation counts. Cornell Lab of Ornithology operates **www.ebird.org** where you can login for free and submit bird lists or find out what's being seen at some of the area's birding hot spots. A similar count is being done for butterflies at **www.wisconsinbutterflies.org/butterflies/sightings.**

- Never spook animals. An unannounced approach, a sudden movement, or a loud noise startles most animals, and a surprised animal can be dangerous. Give them plenty of space.

- Be courteous to others you encounter on the trails.

- Look up! Keep an eye out for standing dead trees and storm-damaged living trees with loose or broken limbs that can fall at any time.

- Know your ability, and carry necessary supplies for changes in weather or other conditions.

TRAIL RECOMMENDATIONS

UP TO 3 MILES

1 Bayside Trail
2 La Jolla: Coast Walk Trail
3 La Jolla Shores: Tide Pools Walk
4 Torrey Pines State Reserve: Guy Fleming Trail
6 Batiquitos Lagoon Trail
8 Inaja Memorial Trail
14 Del Dios Gorge Trail
18 Elfin Forest Recreational Reserve: Botanical Loop
19 Discovery Lake and Hills Loop
21 Los Jilgueros Preserve Trail

3 TO 6 MILES

5 San Elijo Lagoon: La Orilla Trailhead to Rios Avenue Trail
7 Laguna Mountains: Sunset Trail
10 Palomar Mountain: Observatory Trail
11 Lake Morena Trail
12 Miramar Reservoir Loop
15 Lake Poway Loop
16 Blue Sky Trail to Lake Ramona
17 Lake Hodges: North Shore Trail
20 Lake Dixon: Shore View Trail
22 Wilderness Gardens Preserve: Combined Trails Loop

6 TO 8 MILES

9 Santa Ysabel Open Space Preserve East: Kanaka Loop Trail
13 Los Penasquitos Canyon Preserve: West End to Waterfall Loop

DIVERSE HIKES

11 Lake Morena Trail

FAMILY HIKES

4 Torrey Pines State Reserve: Guy Fleming Trail

10 Palomar Mountain: Observatory Trail

21 Los Jilgueros Preserve Trail

22 Wilderness Gardens Preserve: Combined Trails Loop

FLAT HIKES

3 La Jolla Shores: Tide Pools Walk

4 Torrey Pines State Reserve: Guy Fleming Trail

6 Batiquitos Lagoon Trail

14 Del Dios Gorge Trail

17 Lake Hodges: North Shore Trail

21 Los Jilgueros Preserve Trail

HIGH-TRAFFIC HIKES

2 La Jolla: Coast Walk Trail

3 La Jolla Shores: Tide Pools Walk

4 Torrey Pines State Reserve: Guy Fleming Trail

5 San Elijo Lagoon: La Orilla Trailhead to Rios Avenue Trail

7 Laguna Mountains: Sunset Trail

15 Lake Poway Loop

17 Lake Hodges: North Shore Trail

18 Elfin Forest Recreational Reserve: Botanical Loop

20 Lake Dixon: Shore View Trail

HIKES ALONG WATER

3 La Jolla Shores: Tide Pools Walk

4 Torrey Pines State Reserve: Guy Fleming Trail

13 Los Penasquitos Canyon Preserve: West End to Waterfall Loop

17 Lake Hodges: North Shore Trail

18 Elfin Forest Recreational Reserve: Botanical Loop

HIKES FOR BIRDWATCHING

2 La Jolla: Coast Walk Trail
5 San Elijo Lagoon: La Orilla Trailhead to Rios Avenue Trail
6 Batiquitos Lagoon Trail
8 Inaja Memorial Trail
17 Lake Hodges: North Shore Trail
20 Lake Dixon: Shore View Trail

HIKES FOR DOGS

5 San Elijo Lagoon: La Orilla Trailhead to Rios Avenue Trail
8 Inaja Memorial Trail
9 Santa Ysabel Open Space Preserve East: Kanaka Loop Trail
14 Del Dios Gorge Trail
15 Lake Poway Loop
16 Blue Sky Trail to Lake Ramona
17 Lake Hodges: North Shore Trail
18 Elfin Forest Recreational Reserve: Botanical Loop
21 Los Jilgueros Preserve Trail

HIKES FOR VERY YOUNG CHILDREN

3 La Jolla Shores: Tide Pools Walk
11 Lake Morena Trail
18 Elfin Forest Recreational Reserve: Botanical Loop
19 Discovery Lake and Hills Loop

HIKES WITH HISTORICAL INTEREST

1 Bayside Trail
2 La Jolla: Coast Walk Trail
8 Inaja Memorial Trail

HIKES WITH VIEWS

1 Bayside Trail
2 La Jolla: Coast Walk Trail
4 Torrey Pines State Reserve: Guy Fleming Trail

7 Laguna Mountains: Sunset Trail
8 Inaja Memorial Trail

LAKE HIKES

11 Lake Morena Trail
15 Lake Poway Loop
17 Lake Hodges: North Shore Trail
19 Discovery Lake and Hills Loop
20 Lake Dixon: Shore View Trail

LOW-TRAFFIC HIKES

22 Wilderness Gardens Preserve: Combined Trails Loop

MULTIUSE TRAILS

9 Santa Ysabel Open Space Preserve East: Kanaka Loop Trail
13 Los Penasquitos Canyon Preserve: West End to Waterfall Loop
14 Del Dios Gorge Trail
15 Lake Poway Loop
17 Lake Hodges: North Shore Trail

SPRING HIKES FOR WILDFLOWERS

7 Laguna Mountains: Sunset Trail
8 Inaja Memorial Trail
15 Lake Poway Loop

TRAILS FOR RUNNERS

5 San Elijo Lagoon: La Orilla Trailhead to Rios Avenue Trail
6 Batiquitos Lagoon Trail
9 Santa Ysabel Open Space Preserve East: Kanaka Loop Trail
14 Del Dios Gorge Trail
17 Lake Hodges: North Shore Trail

WILDLIFE HIKES

3 La Jolla Shores: Tide Pools Walk
9 Santa Ysabel Open Space Preserve East: Kanaka Loop Trail

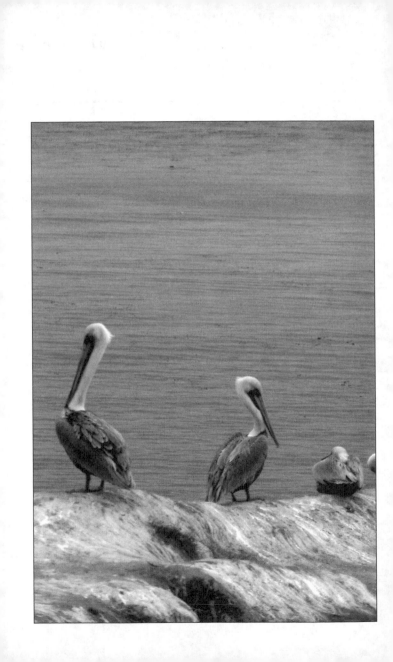

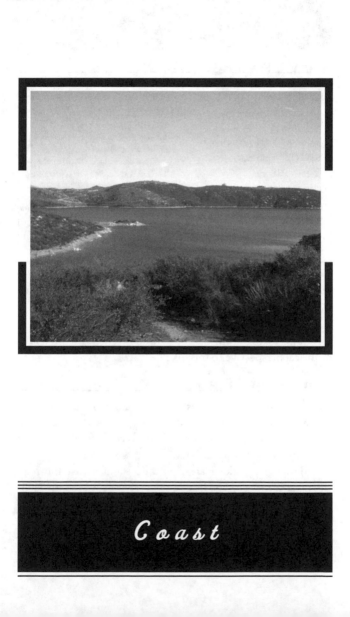

Coast

■ OVERVIEW

LENGTH: 3 miles	**MAPS:** Distributed with parking fee at ranger booth
CONFIGURATION: Out-and-back	
SCENERY: View of San Diego Bay, coastal sage scrub, wildflowers	**FACILITIES:** Restrooms at nearby Cabrillo National Monument Visitor Center and also near the lighthouse; for more information, call (619) 557-5450 or visit the Web site edweb.sdsu.edu/cab.
EXPOSURE: Mostly sunny	
TRAFFIC: Moderate	
TRAIL SURFACE: Gravel	
HIKING TIME: 1.5 hours	**SPECIAL COMMENTS:** Stay close to children on this trail, where cliffs drop to rocky bay shores several hundred feet below in some sections.
ACCESS: $5 car parking fee (free with a National Parks Pass); open 9 a.m.–5 p.m. daily	

■ SNAPSHOT

Cool coastal breezes and sweeping views of San Diego's bay make the Bayside Trail a top choice for warm spring and summer days. Taking in the nearby lighthouse and museum lend a historical perspective to this hike.

■ CLOSE-UP

Its close proximity to the historic Point Loma Lighthouse and the Juan Rodriguez Cabrillo Museum make the Bayside Trail a favorite among energetic tourists. Locals come for the pleasant hike with breathtaking bay views.

From the parking area, proceed south across the road (there's a crosswalk) and head up the sidewalk toward the lighthouse. A sign to the west of the lighthouse indicates the route to the Bayside Trail. Follow this asphalt route down to the southwest for approximately 0.3 miles to the marked trailhead, where there is a bench from which you can see the bay. Foghorns warn sailboats and military vessels to slow down at regular intervals.

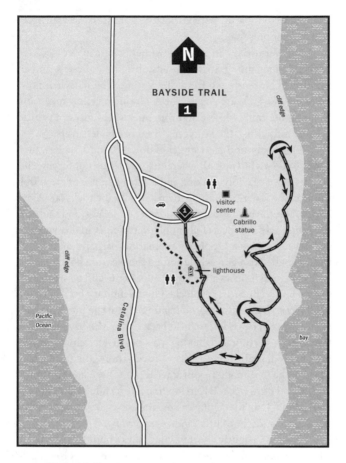

The gravel trail, once used as a military patrol road, gradually descends to the southeast. The valley to your right is furred with thick coastal sage scrub and a grove of mature silver-dollar trees stretching up from the cleft base. On the left, the sandstone cliff rises as the trail descends. Numerous whiptail and Western fence lizards scuttle from open sunning spots into the scrub at the side of the trail. Some will dash across the trail, then pause to look up with curiosity, as if assessing your reaction to their presence.

On warm days in the late winter, one can see signs of spring. Like flaming match heads, bright, coral-red Indian paintbrush blooms peep from the ground. The daisylike flowers of the low-growing encelia shrub bloom in yellow profusion all along the trail, while California buckwheat grows in thick, cottony tufts alongside last year's dried brown leftovers.

This eastbound path stretches down about 0.3 miles, then bends to the right (north), where the trail levels out for a while. You may hear sea lions barking and catch a glimpse of them frolicking in the water or sunning themselves on the rocks far below. Meanwhile, the blue-green water forever undulates, and sailboats of varying sizes bob peacefully or tilt precariously in the wind. It's not unusual to see a U.S. Navy submarine, partially submerged, gliding south like a gray whale among the pleasure boats.

The trail follows a V-shaped inlet in the cliff westward for several hundred yards, past locked metal military bunkers from World War II. Look for a drinking fountain at the point of the V where the trail bears left to head back east to the bay view. The trail swings further left, taking you north for approximately 0.25 miles and affording views of rocky shore, the bright-blue curve of the Coronado Bay Bridge far to the east, and the buildings of downtown San Diego looking like a child's model in the foreground. Don't let children run ahead or get too close to the edge. The sandstone cliffs can be dangerous.

Another, slightly shorter, inlet takes you into a shaded V where toyon and lemonadeberry bushes thrive, growing in thick, man-tall groupings. Wild cucumber vines with delicate white blossoms creep over the smaller shrubs, and tiny hummingbirds hover, moving this way and that. Be careful as the trail heads east toward the bay—the inlet valley isn't as guarded by shrubs on this side.

Along this last stretch of northbound trail, watch for the succulent tubes of the ladyfinger plant along the ground. Also notice the tall, spindly bladderpod and its narrow, pale-green leaves and yellow flowers with protruding stamens. The sweet smell of black sage fills the air. You may also note the tangy-sweet smell of wild licorice. Watch for its pale, fernlike leaves growing on foot-high bushes with vanilla-white blooms.

A sign announces the trail's end (and a chain-link fence several yards past the sign blocks further passage). Follow the trail back the way you came, this time uphill. On hot days, you'll enjoy the shady V inlets as you make the gradual 300-foot climb. Slow down and count the succulent agaves growing on the cliff, or spot the creamy white of a cluster of milkmaids peeking out from beneath the cascading ferns that thrive in the cooler nooks of the inlet trail. If you've taken this hike in the afternoon, look at the silver-dollar trees in the valley to your left as you head west and up toward the trailhead. The trees catch the wind and light, and the leaves sparkle like coins.

■ MORE FUN

Tour the historic Old Point Loma Lighthouse with its spiraling staircase and glassed-in rooms furnished with artifacts and notations that chronicle the lives of the keeper, Robert Israel, and his family. The visitor center offers a museum describing the expeditions of Juan Rodriguez Cabrillo, the first European to set foot on the West Coast of the United States. There is also a gift shop, vending machines, and pay-per-view telescopes for viewing the bay.

■ TO THE TRAILHEAD

From I-5 North or I-8 East, exit at Rosecrans and turn right on Canon, then left on Catalina Boulevard. Follow Catalina Boulevard past Fort Rosecrans Cemetery and drive into the park. Turn left into the well-marked parking area.

02 La Jolla: Coast Walk Trail

■ OVERVIEW

LENGTH: 0.5 miles	**MAPS:** None
CONFIGURATION: Out-and-back or loop	**FACILITIES:** None
SCENERY: Ocean views, birds	**SPECIAL COMMENTS:** Children enjoy this hike, but watch them carefully or insist on holding hands because sheer cliffs that drop 100 feet to the rocky shoreline can be dangerous. Though this hike is enjoyable anytime, fall and winter promise smaller crowds.
EXPOSURE: Mostly sunny	
TRAFFIC: Moderate to heavy	
TRAIL SURFACE: Packed cliffside soil, optional sidewalk add-ons	
HIKING TIME: 30 minutes	
ACCESS: Free	

■ SNAPSHOT

This easy, cliffside walk offers up-close views of dolphins, seals, and resident seabirds. Despite the area's shops and tourism, the habitat of La Jolla's coastline is still a haven for the birds.

■ CLOSE-UP

To the right and left of the cliffside parking spaces on Coast Walk, benches overlooking the ocean offer a spectacular view. Depending on the tide, the waves crash with striking force against the cliffs or gently swell and ebb in a rolling rhythm. The area is popular among kayakers. You may spot them paddling their narrow vessels along the coastline, getting a closer look at the series of watery caves carved into the cliffs below.

The path starts to the left of the parking area, where thick stands of lemonadeberry bushes separate the trail from the cliff's edge. You'll quickly come to a plank bridge and head up wooden steps, reaching an earthen path open to the cliffs. Be careful here, especially with children.

A strong ammonia-like smell may fill the air here. Birds—cormorants, pelicans, and a variety of gulls—are the culprits.

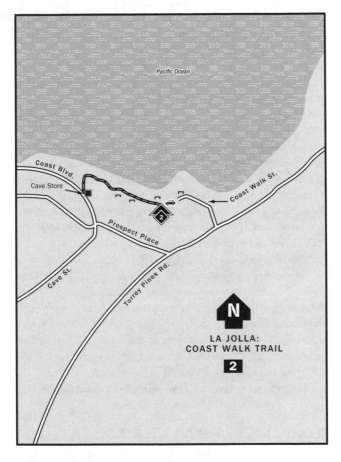

They gather on the rocky cliffs in huge groups—the cormorants clinging to the sides of the steep cliffs, while the gulls and pelicans congregate in groups on the flatter rocks jutting out beyond the path.

Several benches placed along the 0.25-mile-long strip provide opportunities to sit and let the ocean lull you. The strong odor isn't as shocking after a few moments, and it's relaxing to sit here on the brink of the cliffs overlooking the vast watery expanse. The cliffside coast walk is a surprising change of pace from the hustle and bustle of tourist activity along La Jolla's shop-lined streets. But there are other surprises here. You will discover that pelicans may look a bit slow and clumsy on land, but they fly with regal elegance. In large flocks, the graceful-in-flight birds soar toward the coast, surveying the cliffs then doubling back to land among the masses.

A viewing platform near the Cave Street end of the path gets visitors closest to the birds, which gather, preening, on the rocks just a few feet beyond the railing. The clustered birds, the sparkling Pacific Ocean, and the spectacular curving San Diego coastline make this is a favorite spot for photos. You may also spot seals sunning themselves on shoreline rocks below. Even dolphins are a common site in this wonderful coastal nature enclave.

From here, you can exit the path and turn right onto Cave Street, then continue walking along the sidewalk another 0.25 miles or so with pleasant breezes, ocean views, and lovely pathways with embedded shell art. The Children's Pool Beach, where seals gather to give birth to their pups, is just a short distance ahead. Or, instead, turn left, walking up the hill and left again onto Torrey Pines Road, meeting Coast Walk and heading around to your car. If you have the time and energy, do both. Everything is in close proximity here.

■ TO THE TRAILHEAD

Take I-52 West into La Jolla, where it merges into La Jolla Parkway. Continue northwest on La Jolla Parkway for approximately 1 mile, where it becomes Torrey Pines Road. Continue for about 1 more mile and turn right on Coast Walk, a narrow street that holds two cliffside parking spaces a short distance ahead. Because they are hidden, these spaces are often open. If they're in use, turn right back onto Torrey Pines Road. Travel about a 0.1 mile, then turn right again where you see the sign marked "Cave Street."

Park curbside wherever you can—the path's opposite end can be accessed about 200 yards from the junction of Torrey Pines Road, at a grove of pine trees near the Cave Store.

03 La Jolla Shores: Tide Pools Walk

■ OVERVIEW

LENGTH: 2 miles	**MAPS:** None needed
CONFIGURATION: Out-and-back	**FACILITIES:** In the parking area near the lifeguard tower
SCENERY: Ocean waves, tide-pool creatures	**SPECIAL COMMENTS:** Wear sturdy rubber-soled shoes that will cling to wet rock surfaces. You'll need protection to climb among the tide pools. Be sure to visit around low tide. For tide schedules, check www.mobilegeographics.com:81/locations/3220.html.
EXPOSURE: Sunny	
TRAFFIC: Moderate to heavy	
TRAIL SURFACE: Sand and surf, rocks	
HIKING TIME: 1 hour	
ACCESS: Free	

■ SNAPSHOT

The ocean breeze, rolling waves, and sand beneath your feet. Who could ask for more? But that's only the beginning—low tides mean plenty of sea creatures to marvel over.

■ CLOSE-UP

From the grassy area at the north end of Kellogg Park, where free parking is plentiful in the off-season or early on weekday mornings, head north up the beach toward the pier. You might as well kick off your shoes on this wide sandy beach, and let the surf roll in around your feet.

It's about 0.5 miles to the pier that extends from UCSD's Scripps Institute of Oceanography on the cliff above the beach (the cliff and the institute are not open to the public). Standing

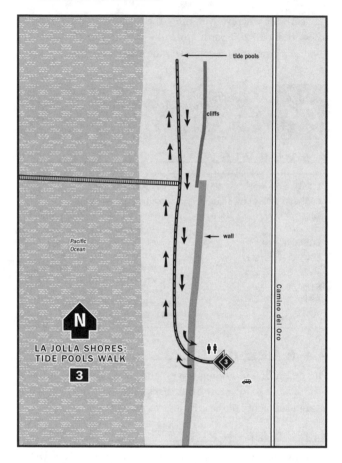

beneath the pier between the wide mussel-encrusted supports, one can only marvel at man's ability to build structures strong enough to withstand the ocean's power. A short distance ahead, though, tiny creatures thrive in the ocean's ebb and flow— proving worthy design on a small scale.

As you continue north you'll see more and more large rocks, pitted by the sea and sand, strewn along the beach. Stuff your feet back into shoes to cross a strip of piled, rounded rocks that form a hobbling path near the base of the cliffs. The larger rocks, roughened into various shapes by wind, water, and sand, clump together, leaving little sand between them.

As you hop from rock to rock, startled crabs scurry sideways into crevices. Schools of fish trapped in pools left by the receding tide swim to safety among fluttery pink and mauve sea plants. Take the time to stoop and get a closer look at what may seem at first just an empty pool. Often, you'll discover that the collected water teems with life.

Squabbling over territory, hermit crabs scuttle about in temporary shell houses that are sometimes smaller than a pea. The bigger crabs carry larger shells. Notice the variety of shapes and sizes they select. Even a broken shell may be chosen by a less discerning hermit crab; as he haltingly makes his way across the waterscape, the shell's uneven edge catches on everything he passes. A rusty-colored sea plant suddenly moves away, and you realize it's a sea slug. Watch for a moment and see several more that have been camouflaged in plain sight advance into view. Clumps of elongated oval mussels adhere to the rocks. Sea anemones contract when touched. Gently touching the animals is permitted, but you may not collect or remove anything from the area.

From the rocky tide pool area, you could hike about 3.5 more miles to Flat Rock, named for its shape, and access a climbing route ("Beach Trail") up into Torrey Pines State Reserve. You may spot nude sunbathers along the way: past the rocky tidepools is the area called "Black's Beach," well known as a clothing-optional zone—although public nudity is illegal.

■ MORE FUN

If the tide pools have whet your appetite for knowledge about the ocean and its wildlife, the nearby Birch Aquarium at 2300 Expedition Way in La Jolla is worth a visit. Consult the facility's

Web site at **www.aquarium.ucsd.edu** or call (858) 534-3474 for more information.

■ TO THE TRAILHEAD

From CA 52 West, merge onto La Jolla Parkway, drive 1.4 miles, and turn right on Calle de la Plata. Continue 0.2 miles to Avenida de la Playa and turn left. Drive 0.1 mile to Camino del Oro and spot the park. Drive to the north end of the parking area and park near the lifeguard tower and restrooms.

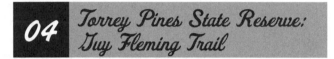

04   Torrey Pines State Reserve: Guy Fleming Trail

■ OVERVIEW

LENGTH: 0.7 miles

CONFIGURATION: Balloon and string

SCENERY: Sweeping ocean views, wildlife, intricate cliff erosion

EXPOSURE: Mostly exposed to sun, but with some shady areas

TRAFFIC: Moderate to heavy

TRAIL SURFACE: Puddles after rain, well-maintained sandy soil paths

HIKING TIME: 30 minutes to 1 hour

ACCESS: Day-use fee to park ($6 weekdays, $8 weekends for automobiles; senior and disabled discounts; additional fees for buses); open daily 8 a.m. until sunset (visitor center opens at 9 a.m.)

MAPS: Download at www.torrey pine.org/activities/hiking-trails.htm or obtain at the park.

FACILITIES: Restrooms located in the upper parking lot

SPECIAL COMMENTS: No food or pets are allowed in this serene, coastal clifftop setting above the ocean. Trails are reserved for foot traffic only. Arrive in time to see the sun slipping into the horizon, painting the sky brilliant orange, dusky purple, or flamingo pink. To extend this easy hike, you may opt to park in free stalls along the beach (as crowds permit), or in the lower lot behind the ranger booth, then walk the approximate 1 uphill mile to the Guy Fleming trailhead.

■ SNAPSHOT

No hurrying allowed—fill your senses with the serenity of nature's power and beauty during an easy stroll along the Guy

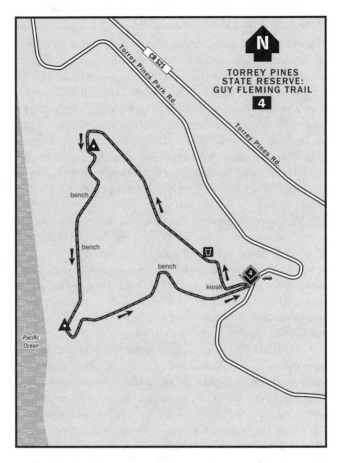

Fleming Trail. Puffy, gilt-edged clouds drift overhead, and a refreshing breeze guides you along the meandering path to ocean overlooks. Bring binoculars—you can often spot dolphins in the waters below. Also watch for migrating whales during the winter viewing season, or just let your mind wander as you sit on one of the many benches, letting the roar of the ocean lull you.

■ **C L O S E - U P**

Enter the Guy Fleming Trail just as Torrey Pines Park Road curves sharply west. You'll find a kiosk with information just a few short steps into the trail, and the loop opens to the right or left. Either way is fun. Go right to follow along with this description. The trail moves northwest at a very slight climb, quickly passing by a drinking fountain and rounding the bend into shade, where northeast views offer glimpses through the pines of Los Penasquitos Lagoon far below. The water stretches out amid the marshy land like dark, abstractly shaped mirrors reflecting the sky. On the right, you'll catch glimpses of La Jolla, etched against the sky and sea.

As the path curves to the west, you may need to duck in places. Twisty limbs of mature Torrey pines hang over the trail. At 0.25 miles, the path moves out of the forest, and an unobstructed view of the Pacific Ocean rolls out before you: glassy, foamy-green, gray, or blue, the water's ever-changing (yet always beautiful) nature makes frequent visits to this easy path a must. Step down to the northernmost overlook point, where a bench perches you cliffside for a gull's-eye view.

From here, surf and sea mesmerize. Drink in the clear salt air, ponder the ocean's ominous power, or reflect on the softest whisper of a gentle breeze against your cheek. Benches rest at regular intervals along this western ridge, leading to another lookout point down some wooden steps to the right of the trail. You'll have come about 0.5 miles at this point, so reward yourself with a long pause . . . the ocean calls, its roaring rhythm like calming white noise.

North and south, the shore stretches for miles. Beachcombers move along like ants on the sand far below, and the waves decorate the shore with lacy foam they leave in their wake.

Eventually, perhaps as the fiery sphere of the sun dips beyond the horizon, head back up the stairs, and to the right on the trail, moving east, away from the coast. You may see quail, curious squirrels, or perhaps a raven or two. Regardless, you're sure to wear a relaxed and ready smile—returned by passersby as you continue along the path, closing the loop back at the kiosk and returning the way you came on this magical little trip into nature's beauty.

■ TO THE TRAILHEAD

From I-5, exit on Carmel Valley Road and drive west for about 1.5 miles till you reach the Coast Highway 101 (US 101). Turn left and proceed along the beach for about 1 mile. The park entrance is on your right just before the highway begins to climb the Torrey Pines grade. Parking choices include a small roadside area just outside the Guy Fleming Loop, a larger upper lot near the visitor center, the lower lot, or free parking along the beach (which adds to your hike; see Special Comments).

05 San Elijo Lagoon: La Orilla Trailhead to Rios Avenue Trail

■ OVERVIEW

LENGTH: 6.7 miles

CONFIGURATION: Out-and-back

SCENERY: Birds, coastal sage scrub, lagoon waters

EXPOSURE: Sunny

TRAFFIC: Moderate to heavy

TRAIL SURFACE: Packed and soft sand

HIKING TIME: 2.5 to 3 hours

ACCESS: Free

MAPS: Call (760) 436-3944, or view online at www.sanelijo.org

FACILITIES: None

SPECIAL COMMENTS: This is an ecological preserve. Leashed dogs only; owners must pick up after them. Although not a traditional horse park where riders trailer in their horses, people from the surrounding area do sometimes ride here. No bicycling is allowed. For more information, visit www.sanelijo.org.

■ SNAPSHOT

This easy stroll through nature is popular with families, walkers, and joggers. People often bring their dogs (on leashes) here.

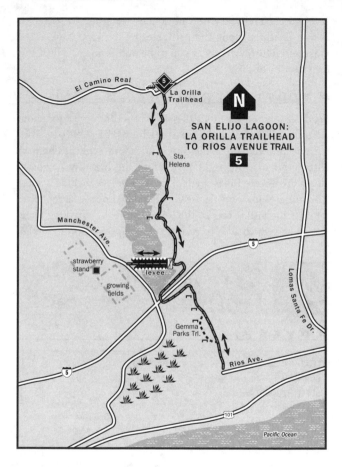

El Camino Real

La Orilla
Trailhead

N

**SAN ELIJO LAGOON:
LA ORILLA TRAILHEAD
TO RIOS AVENUE TRAIL**

5

Sta.
Helena

Manchester Ave

strawberry
stand

growing
fields

levee

Gemma
Parks Trl.

Rios Ave.

Lomas Santa Fe Dr.

Pacific Ocean

■ CLOSE-UP

From the trailhead, proceed west past the entry kiosk through eucalyptus forest, where a variety of toadstools call the moist path home. Hummingbirds buzz in the branches overhead. The younger, spindly trees grow close together here. Their branches chafe one another in the breeze, making a squeaking noise that may have you wondering if an unusual bird is in the treetops.

At 0.2 miles, the trail moves out of the trees. Lemonadeberry, toyon, prickly-pear cactus, bladderpod, and scrub oak line the path. Creeping wild cucumber vines twine over the bushes like a lacy veil. At about 0.4 miles, cross the Sta. Helena side trail and continue. Mature pine trees spot the land as the trail gradually climbs. The lagoon soon comes into view on the right, about 50 yards from the path. There are always ducks here, paddling about in pairs. You might also see egrets, herons, and a variety of other birds—295 species have been spotted here at San Elijo Lagoon.

As you continue, sweeping views of the lagoon alternate with areas where thick toyon, sumac, and scrub oak rim the trail. White and black sage grows here, emitting a refreshing scent. The red and yellow of California fuchsia and fiddleweed provide bright splotches of color.

At about 0.7 miles, a side trail loops off to the right. Follow it across a level plain that moves closer to the water. The path comes to an overlook point with a bench, then heads south and reconnects with the main trail. Go right, continuing west on the main trail. Ice plant grows in the soft sand that slows you down here.

At 1.5 miles, the trail bears right. Head around the chainlink pass-through for access to the concrete levee. Sometimes the concrete levee is dry, and other times (seasonally), the water trickles over the cement. Bird tracks of varying shapes and sizes form interesting patterns on the cement. Ducks paddle in and out of the marsh alongside the levee as herons and egrets wade and feed in the shallows. The levee trail ends after 0.3 miles, where it reaches Manchester Avenue. Double back to the pass-through and continue. Pass the point where you turned right to reach the levee. Continue southwest for a short distance and bear right where the trail makes a U-turn, then walk parallel to I-5 on the left for 0.25 miles or so.

At the interstate overpass, follow a narrow trail leading under the freeway and emerge on the west side of I-5, where there is a high trail and a low trail. Both trails head south, paralleling the freeway for about 0.2 miles. Runners seem to favor the high trail, which is separated from the low trail by a sandbar that cushions the sound of the highway traffic. If you choose the low one, notice the millions of shells filling the sand, which has piled high on the left as the water has filled the trail and receded. Pickleweed grows along this stretch that heads west through eucalyptus and willow forest. At 2.7 miles from the trailhead, you'll reach a wooden bench that faces the bird-filled marsh.

From here, the trail bends west. You'll find another bench just ahead. Continue west for another 1 mile, where the trail forks right to continue along the lagoon edge. This segment is called the Gemma Parks Interpretive Trail. You'll find more benches facing the lagoon along this stretch. Marsh plants grow low, which is good for bird-watching. The Gemma Parks Trail soon junctions the main route again. Turning right takes you another 0.2 miles to Rios Avenue. Some hikers choose to begin the hike at the Rios Avenue trailhead, taking the trail from the opposite end.

■ MORE FUN

When visiting the levee in summer, you may notice growing fields across Manchester Avenue. A strawberry stand there sells the sweet, juicy produce.

■ TO THE TRAILHEAD

Take I-5 to the Lomas Santa Fe Road exit. Head east for about 1 mile to Highland Road, then turn left. After about 0.5 miles, turn left on El Camino Real. Drive 0.5 miles; the trail entrance is on the left. Park in the dirt area adjacent to El Camino Real.

OVERVIEW

LENGTH: 3 miles

CONFIGURATION: Out-and-back

SCENERY: Native sage scrub, birds and their nesting sites

EXPOSURE: Sunny and shady

TRAFFIC: Heavy

TRAIL SURFACE: Sandy soil

HIKING TIME: 1 hour

ACCESS: Free

MAPS: At the Batiquitos Lagoon Foun-dation Web site, www.batiquitos foundation.org or the restoration Web site, www.batiquitos.org

FACILITIES: Restroom at the nature center

SPECIAL COMMENTS: The nature center offers guided walks and lots of learning opportunities. The trail does not allow bikes or horses. For more information, see the foundation's Web site or call (760) 931-0800.

SNAPSHOT

Cool ocean breezes and glassy water that laps soothingly at the shore make this a refreshing hike for hotter days, and the trail is easy. Bring your children for an educational experience, including a visit to the nature center, where friendly guides enjoy sharing information.

CLOSE-UP

Walk southeast on the paved section; you quickly come to the nature center. There, colorful seabird cutouts offer still-life clues as to what you're likely to see in full living color ahead—birds, birds, and more birds—grebes, herons, plovers, terns, and more.

Just past the nature center, the dirt trail begins. The lagoon waters gently lap the shore to the right of the path while, beyond it, the freeway incessantly hums. Concentrate on the birds floating along where the ripples take them or ducking their heads beneath the glassy water in search of food. Slow-winged gulls sail along on the air. Drawing your attention to the

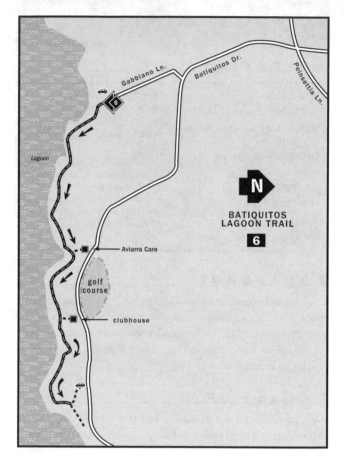

moment, the yellow-beaked gulls seem to carry the traffic noise away on their lazy flight.

Information panels offer facts about surrounding marsh vegetation, like the fleshy pickleweed, rustling cattail, heath, or salt grass. Look closely amid the greenery: a plover rests atop a stick in the mud, and an egret stands so still he seems to be a part of the landscape.

Benches are placed approximately every third of a mile and overlook the lagoon the same way several houses on the left do, poised to enjoy the rippling water through south-facing windows shaded against the afternoon sun—or perhaps thrown open to allow in the musky scent of thriving coastal sage scrub.

The route bears left through eucalyptus trees with trunks that creak and squeak as the wind pushes them against each other. Note Aviarra Cove on the left (another entrance to the lagoon) and continue east. A golf course appears, with its man-icured grass looking almost artificial against this natural setting. Two worlds usually so far apart collide here, where golfers in collared shirts wave at hikers in boots or running shoes. Look up into the trees as you head through this section. Guides tell of great blue herons nesting overhead year after year.

Another quarter of a mile or so brings you past the golf clubhouse and then to the eastern entrance, which is a good place to turn around. You'll notice a protected nesting area for the threatened snowy plover and endangered least tern. Be sure to visit during nesting season, generally from May to August.

Enjoy the fresh coastal air and absorb the ever-changing palette of nature's canvas as you retrace your steps. The late-afternoon sun forms stripes on the lagoon waters as though fil-tered through blinds.

■ TO THE TRAILHEAD

Take I-5 to the Poinsettia Lane exit and drive 0.3 miles east to Batiquitos Drive. Turn right and continue 0.4 miles to where the road curves southwest. Turn right on Gabbiano Lane and drive 0.3 miles to the parking lot at the trailhead.

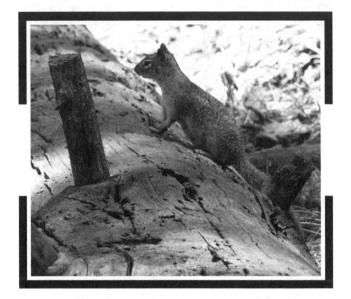

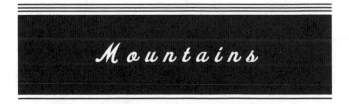

Mountains

■ OVERVIEW

LENGTH: 3 miles

CONFIGURATION: Out-and-back

SCENERY: Forest, water, birds

EXPOSURE: Filtered and full sun

TRAFFIC: Moderate

TRAIL SURFACE: Earthen path, some rocky areas

HIKING TIME: 1.5 hours

ACCESS: Parked vehicles must display an "Adventure Pass," sold at the visitor center or at the Mount Laguna Lodge Store located about 8 miles north of I-8 on Sunrise Highway. For more information, call (619) 473-8547 or visit www.lmva.org.

MAPS: Available for purchase at the

visitor center, online at www.lmva.org, at the Lodge Store, and at the Blue Jay Restaurant; see www.lmva.org or www.lagunamountain.com for more information.

FACILITIES: None

SPECIAL COMMENTS: The thin air at nearly 6,000 feet can make this easy hike seem slightly longer than the measured mileage. Occasionally, winter snow closes the Sunset Highway (a.k.a. County Route S1) or makes tire chains necessary. For current conditions, call the California Highway Patrol at (858) 637-3800 or check the "traffic incidents" section at cad.chp.ca.gov.

■ SNAPSHOT

This fairly short route to the water in the woods is only a portion of the Sunset Trail but provides a quick, quiet interlude with nature and all its stress-relieving qualities. Squirrels abound on this parklike hike without the pavement, joggers, or city commotion. Before you start, consider applying an insect repellent to combat biting flies.

■ CLOSE-UP

The narrow trail starts off heading north through meadowland and toward trees, climbing ever so gradually. The path is reserved for foot traffic, but you may notice (thankfully only a few) bicycle tire tracks. After a few steps, you'll come to a trail split; go left toward water in the woods.

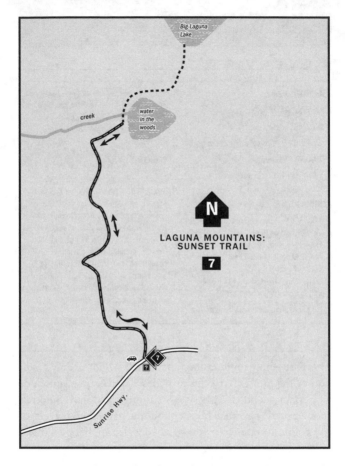

At around 0.4 miles, the trail comes to a ridge overlooking distant, golden meadows. Early mornings mean a view of the clouds settling over the valley. Later, the setting sun's rays spill orange and pink into the dusky sky. There's a rocky area along this section, but nothing difficult. Some large boulders provide resting spots for those who wish to pause and appreciate the views.

Turning right takes you to a meadow dotted with trees, thick in places. Beware of biting flies wanting to make a meal of exposed skin. In the spring you'll see a variety of butterflies flitting from flower to flower—pale purple fleabane with its yellow center, bright-scarlet bugler and Indian paintbrush, sunny golden yarrow, and an array of others.

Disturbed by hikers' feet, a multitude of dull grasshoppers lying camouflaged in the dirt open their wings to reveal the vibrant orange. Fluttering away, they sound like shaking maracas.

At about 0.6 miles, the trail moves fairly steeply downhill, into black oak forest. The steep section is short and not so vertical that you must slow down. A more gradual descent stretches about a third of a mile farther. The trail then levels for a bit before climbing upward through thicker forest. The shade casts shadows, and rocks sticking up in the path might go unseen: watch your step as you pick your way through the woods.

When you come to an outcropping of rocks on the right and the path crosses the flat edge of a boulder, you'll know you've nearly reached the pond. The trail opens to a wide meadow, revealing a seasonal creek to the left just ahead. The pond teems with life. A variety of algae provides hiding places for aquatic bugs; birds come for a drink and dragonflies buzz about, then rest atop the scummy floating pads of algae.

If you want to go farther, an additional 0.5 miles or so leads to Big Laguna Lake (but thanks to drought, you can't count on the presence of water). Go left past the pond and head north to reach the lake. The Sunset Trail also continues to the north side of the lake, allowing you to connect to other trails for a long loop if you prefer (consult the Mount Laguna area map).

Otherwise, sit on a log overlooking the pond. If you brought lunch, count on squirrels to pay a visit, hoping for a handout. Enjoy the reflection of the trees on the water's blue-green surface, breathe in the fresh scent of the mountain air, and relax before retracing your steps back to the highway and your car.

■ TO THE TRAILHEAD

From I-8, take the Sunset Highway exit, turn left (north), and drive 5.1 miles. You'll spot an observation deck and call box on the right; park on the shoulder (where there is plenty of room). The trailhead is across the street, a few hundred feet north.

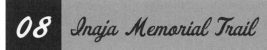

08 Inaja Memorial Trail

■ OVERVIEW

LENGTH: 0.6 miles round-trip	by numbered poles at: www.fs.fed .us/r5/cleveland/recreation/trails/ inaja.shtml
CONFIGURATION: Balloon and string	
SCENERY: Views of Santa Ysabel Valley, surrounding landmarks	**FACILITIES:** Vault-style restrooms, picnic sites with bench tables and barbecues
EXPOSURE: Open to sun	
TRAFFIC: Light on weekdays, moderate to heavy on weekends	**SPECIAL COMMENTS:** An easy stop-off point for travelers, the trail is heavily used on weekends, often by dog-walkers (leashed allowed). Steeper points may be slippery, so appropriately soled shoes and a walking stick are useful.
TRAIL SURFACE: Silty soil	
HIKING TIME: 20–30 minutes	
ACCESS: Free	
MAPS: None known. Find a printable online guide to the plants marked	

■ SNAPSHOT

Beauty surrounds you on every foot of this short trail. Oaks, birds, hulking lichen-speckled boulders, and sweeping views exist at every turn. Birdsong, a gentle breeze, and the scents of spring flowers and pines engage the senses.

■ CLOSE-UP

From the parking lot, walk east toward the kiosk and onto the narrow asphalt path that leads past the stone memorial on the

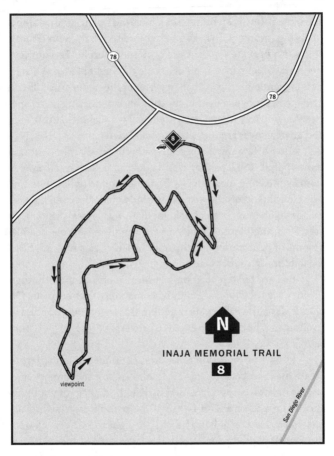

INAJA MEMORIAL TRAIL
8

viewpoint

San Diego River

right, and into several picnic spots among the trees. This site was dedicated to 11 men who lost their lives fighting a 1956 Inaja forest fire. The paved path curves right, past the restrooms, and then the pavement ends, opening to an earthen trail.

Immediately upon stepping onto the leaf-littered course, enchantment abounds. Particularly in the moderate seasons, the area is alive with color, scent, and sound. Lichen forms elaborate patterns on boulders as you head up the gradual slope. In spring, monkey flowers greet you with coral-colored faces, and salvia provides splashes of blooming purple. To your left, the forest opens into a golden valley. A red-tailed hawk may soar on gentle breezes. Quail may run in the underbrush. If you love birds, binoculars aid in spotting and identifying many species you're likely to see here. Steller's Jays, California towhees, and gnatcatchers are just a few possibilities.

After a few short steps the path curves sharply right and moves uphill. You'll pass by a left-hand trail (which you'll emerge from later having made the loop) and continue uphill. The trail bears left and opens to sweeping westerly views between the lush foliage of mature oaks. Look for native chamise dripping in creamy spring blooms. Golden yarrow and the purple bell-like blooms of penstemon line the trail, which climbs upward, bearing left through a rocky section to the viewpoint.

Be sure to step atop the platform rock and look through the viewing tube for area landmarks marked on a steel plate. On cloudy days, the valleys surrounding this point are shrouded in a rolling fog, but on clear days the proverbial "forever" is within sight.

From this high point, the trail continues bending left to create the loop back down. The path can be a bit slippery on a couple of short steep areas. Stay safe with the help of a walking stick, and take care with footing. The path intersects with the one you started on at half a mile. Turn right and head back onto the asphalt path, through the picnic area and past the memorial monument. Back at the kiosk near the parking lot, you'll have traveled 0.6 miles, refreshed from a gentle sample of the Cleveland National Forest.

■ MORE FUN

Head back into the town of Julian and stop to stroll the peaceful streets, poke your head into some of the quaint shops and eateries, or enjoy a horse and carriage ride on Main Street. On weekends, tourists sometimes jam the town, but quiet weekdays foster a slower pace of yesteryear.

■ TO THE TRAILHEAD

Take I-8 East to CA 79 and travel north past Lake Cuyamaca (about 10 miles) into the town of Julian, then head west through the town for just a short distance. Where Main Street intersects CA 78, turn left. Drive approximately 5 miles. Inaja Memorial Park is on the left, with ample parking.

09 Santa Ysabel Open Space Preserve East: Kanaka Loop Trail

■ OVERVIEW

LENGTH: Approximately 7 miles round-trip

CONFIGURATION: Balloon and string

SCENERY: Possible wildlife sightings, rolling hills, oak forest

EXPOSURE: Sun and shade

TRAFFIC: Moderate

TRAIL SURFACE: Packed soil, can be muddy after rain or snow

HIKING TIME: 2.5 to 3 hours

ACCESS: Free; open 7 days, 8 a.m.–7 p.m. during daylight savings time, and 8 a.m.–5 p.m. during standard time

MAPS: Viewable on kiosk near gate, or for download at www.co.san-diego .ca.us/parks/media/SantaYsabel_ Trails.pdf

FACILITIES: None

SPECIAL COMMENTS: Leashed dogs are allowed on this wide multiuse trail that's fast becoming a popular equestrian spot. As of spring 2007, the fences between the preserve and neighboring reservation lands needed repair. The result: you may encounter cattle that have roamed into the preserve, which has a total of 11 miles of trail.

■ SNAPSHOT

Open to the public since the fall of 2006, these road-width trails through sweeping grasslands, rolling hills, and oak forest

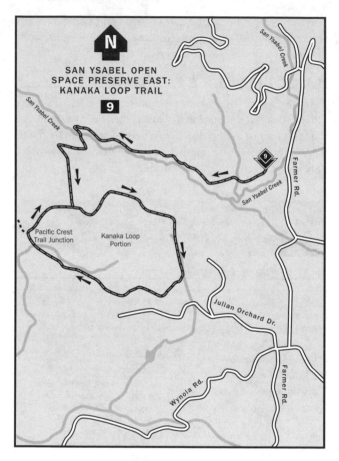

require little analysis. Bring along a friend for a leisurely stroll spent chatting, or a brisk race-walk on a well-kept route covering 7 miles.

■ CLOSE-UP

Head past the kiosk and onto the trail, which begins moving easily through the rolling grassland hills typical of the Santa

Ysabel area. You'll cross the seasonal stream at approximately 0.2 miles, and continue along the westerly route. Watch for cattle from neighboring reservation lands, which, as of this writing, may still be entering the preserve through fences in disrepair. At 0.65 miles, an information panel describes how wildfires can affect the landscape. A patch of oaks provides shade just past the panel, and the creek runs on lower ground to the left of the trail. Wild turkeys are a common sight. Approximately 50 made their way up the hillside on a recent visit. In spring, the males spread their tail feathers and strut noisily about, competing for the attention of the smaller females.

At approximately 1.5 miles, the trail bends left, leading to a shaded picnic bench, then crosses the stream again. From here, the trail moves upward through scrub oaks to a second wildfire information panel at 1.75 miles. The route then bends left, moving steeply uphill for about 0.25 miles. At 2.15 miles, you'll come to a junction. Head left, continuing onto the Kanaka Loop. The trail will descend a little, with evidence of recent fires showing on the remaining area pines. The path climbs steadily for about 0.3 miles. Take your time and enjoy the quiet and wide-open spaces of this preserve that is so true to its name. The sky seems to go on forever above the expanse of rolling grasslands.

A long southerly stretch eventually bends west at approximately 3.3 miles, climbing for a short distance before descending in a long, gradual stretch that levels into a wide, grassy valley. Listen for the calls of birds and enjoy the whisper of rustling grass and breezes. At 4.3 miles, you'll cross the creek again and then reach the junction of the Coast to Crest Trail and this loop. The Coast to Crest Trail extends approximately 2 miles, reaching the West Vista Loop Trail at the west end of the preserve; you might want to try that path another day. For now, pass through the junction, moving 0.33 miles northeast back to where you entered the loop from the main trail. On clear days, you can see the white cap of Palomar Observatory in the northern distance from here. Retrace your steps back down the hill, past the shaded picnic bench and out of the preserve, for a total of 7 miles of easy strolling through this beautiful and peaceful addition to San Diego's public lands.

■ MORE FUN

Apple orchards thrive in Julian. Try the Julian Pie Company for a taste of local apples in America's favorite pie. For more information, visit **www.julianpie.com.**

■ TO THE TRAILHEAD

Take I-8 East to the Japatul/CA 79 exit and turn left. Drive 2.5 miles and turn left onto CA 79 north toward Julian. Continue on CA 79 for approximately 21 miles, to where the road comes to a T. Turn left on Main Street and head through the town of Julian. Main Street becomes Farmer Street after passing through town (less than a mile). After 2.2 miles, turn right onto Wynola Road, travel 100 yards, then turn left onto Farmer Road. Pass the Volcan Mountain Wilderness Preserve sign on your right, and continue approximately 1 mile to the large staging area for Santa Ysabel Open Space Preserve, on the left.

Palomar Mountain: Observatory Trail

■ OVERVIEW

LENGTH: 3.8 miles round-trip

CONFIGURATION: Out-and-back

SCENERY: Pine–oak woodland, possible wildlife, valley views, observatory

EXPOSURE: Mostly dappled shade

TRAFFIC: Light–moderate

TRAIL SURFACE: Leaf-littered; some rocky areas

HIKING TIME: 2 hours

ACCESS: The trail is part of the Cleveland National Forest, so you will need an Adventure Pass to park. You can buy the pass directly from the U.S.

Forest Service online (www.fs.fed .us/r5/sanbernardino/ap) or at the nearby general store. A National Parks and Federal Recreational Lands Annual Pass is also acceptable. Open May–November.

MAPS: None

FACILITIES: Restrooms near parking area

SPECIAL COMMENTS: Dress for the fickle mountain weather, bring plenty of water, and wear boots with good traction for possible snow, mud, or running water. Watch closely for rattlesnakes.

■ SNAPSHOT

If you're looking for woodland splendor and quietude, you'll get instant gratification here. Just a few steps from the trailhead, a dense oak-and-conifer forest envelops you.

■ CLOSE-UP

The narrow, well-defined trail moves northeast, gradually but steadily gaining elevation (about 900 feet in the first mile). I've described the difficulty level as moderate, mainly because the hike begins at nearly 4,500 feet above sea level, and higher altitude, with its thinner air, makes physical activity more difficult. Plenty of benches are placed in shady resting spots along the path. You'll come to the first one just 0.3 miles into the outing.

In spring, you're likely to see lots of blooms—fleabane, goldenrod, and yellow monkey flower, to name a few—in spots

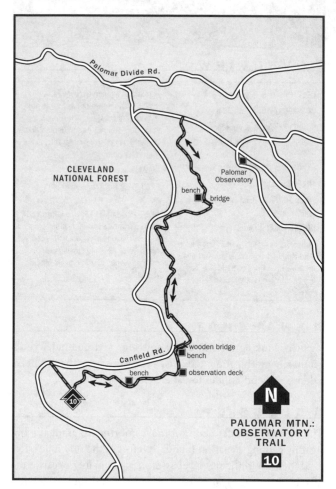

where dappled sunlight filters in through the stretching limbs of mature oaks and pines. Be wary of poison oak, which you'll likely encounter here wherever there's plentiful shade and ample moisture due to snowmelt. Stay on this trail and watch for straying branches of the plant, which sometimes encroach on the path.

At just under 0.6 miles, an observation deck to the right of the trail overlooks lovely Mendenhall Valley. In summer, the golden meadow, dotted with small bodies of water and framed by pines, looks like the proverbial vacation postcard. In other seasons, new spring growth, fall's colors, or pure-white snow makes the view a perfect greeting-card photo.

A few more steps forward bring you to a wooden-plank bridge traversing a gorge that carries seasonal watershed. Manzanita grows more prevalently along this stretch, its deep red bark contrasting with its pale, blue-green leaves. Forest shade is thicker here, too. Just 0.2 miles ahead, find another bench parked among the trees. Relish the cooler temperature here among the protective leaf cover. Some large boulders add interest. Lichen and moss decorating the large rocks bear witness to the random beauty of nature's patterns.

The trail descends along a shaded hillside. A massive seven-trunked oak stands to the left of the trail, which bends more due north at this point. Water runs in the ravine below on your right, a gurgling complement to the soothing lull of the breeze—or perhaps the unwelcome buzz of flying insects. As is the case in many mountain areas, flies and gnats can get troublesome during summer weather. A netted face cover may help.

The path begins to climb again, fresh pine scenting the air. In wetter months, you may find yourself slogging through snow, mud, or water. In drier months, you'll see evidence of moisture: rocks are stained white with water-borne minerals, and a few spiky rushes grow among the stones.

At just under 1 mile, the trail switches abruptly right (east), then back again. The path opens to sunlight for a short stretch, with CA S6 visible 6 to 700 yards away on the left. Come to a bench at a little more than a mile, where the shade begins again. Other than a couple of small hills and dales, the trail remains level for about 0.3 miles. A brief climb meanders east, then north, then east again through dense oak forest above CA S6. In late afternoon, the breezes draft up the through the trees, the rushing sound a reminder of nature's power. The trail dips again, and you'll notice the moon-white cap of Palomar Observatory peeking through the trees. Watch your step, as some fallen trees may have companions helping you up or perhaps teasing, "How was your trip?" Also be mindful of profuse poison oak along this stretch—which may trip up your comfort later.

A small plank bridge crosses a stream at just under 1.7 miles; then the trail gradually climbs again, to a shaded bench.

At 1.9 miles (per my GPS, 2.2 miles on the National Forest map at the trail's end), the path ends abruptly alongside the endpoint for CA S6. Here, at 5,500 feet, you can make your way through the parking lot and visit the observatory (see More Fun, below). Or head back the way you came, moving quickly along on the now mostly downhill path.

■ MORE FUN

Palomar Observatory, a pleasant diversion midhike, is open daily from 9 a.m. to 4 p.m. For more information, call (760) 742-2119 or visit **astro.caltech.edu/palomarnew.**

■ TO THE TRAILHEAD

Take I-15 to the CA 76 exit and head east (inland). Drive approximately 20.4 miles and note a road forking northeast off to the left (marked "South Grade"). Go left onto this road and continue northeast for 6.5 miles where you will come to a T. Turn left here, onto CA S6 and drive approximately 3 miles to the Palomar Observatory Campground entrance on the right. Turn in and follow the campground loop to a small turnout lot (signed) near camp spaces 19 and 20.

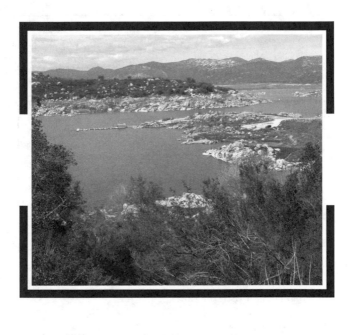

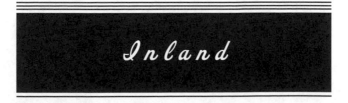

Inland

■ OVERVIEW

LENGTH: 4.8 miles

CONFIGURATION: Out-and-back

SCENERY: View of lake, pine and oak forest

EXPOSURE: Partially shaded

TRAFFIC: Light

TRAIL SURFACE: Packed soil

HIKING TIME: 3.5 hours

ACCESS: $2 per car parking fee

MAPS: Distributed with parking fee at ranger booth, or available online at www.co.san-diego.ca.us/parks/Camping/lake_morena_map.html

FACILITIES: Restrooms in campground area

SPECIAL COMMENTS: Watch for snakes, including rattlesnakes; the wide-open space of the trail makes for good observation. If you have small children, stay safe and skip the high, narrow Hauser Overlook Trail section; remain on the wide main trail, where even pushing a stroller is possible. For information, call (858) 565-3600.

■ SNAPSHOT

This pleasant hike through varying landscapes offers view after view of postcard-perfect scenery that makes the 60-mile drive from San Diego worth the time.

■ CLOSE-UP

From the small dirt lot, walk back around to the gate you passed to park. Access a southwest-bound dirt road, Ward's Flat Trail, partially shaded by cottonwood trees on the right. The route curves, traveling around a finger of Lake Morena, and begins to head northwest. Outcroppings of lichen-encrusted granite rise on the left, some like sheer walls with oak trees seemingly growing right from their craggy faces. Birdsong fills the air.

At 0.7 miles, a granite step stretches out on the right, creating a natural balcony overlooking Lake Morena that is framed by the gnarled branches of an old knotty oak. The trail climbs very gradually past Indian paintbrush growing in fiery, coral-red

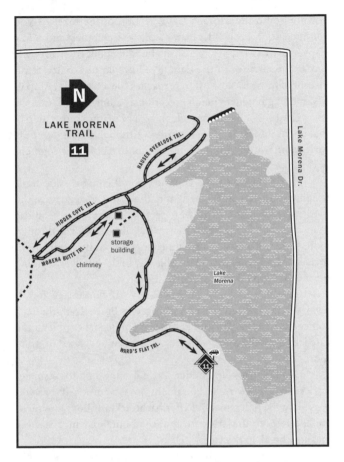

clumps; boulder walls soon give way to flat meadows. In spring, yellow daisylike flowers no bigger than your fingertip carpet the ground and emit a nearly suffocating tangy-sweet scent.

At about 1 mile you'll notice the connecting trail on the right. Pass it for now; also pass the short, dead-end road on the left that leads to a dilapidated metal storage barn. The trail curves south, heading away from the lake, and moves slightly downhill onto the Morena Butte section of the hike. As you continue, look for a dilapidated concrete chimney and a few steps—all that's left of a recreation building built some 80 years ago. In the distance to the right, a red-brown rock butte, reminiscent of those in New Mexico, reaches toward the sky. Atop it, freestanding boulders perch precariously along the ridge.

Continue hiking through an area of mature pine and oak that opens into wide, grassy prairies. Although the landscape is varied, the towering pines lend an alpine feel to this segment of the hike.

Half a mile past the chimney, you'll come to side trails heading southeast and west. Ignore these and, instead, turn the corner to reach the northwest section of the Morena Butte Trail, making your way back toward the lake. You'll pass through more towering pines and spot a connecting trail on your right that leads back to Ward's Flat Trail. Stay to the left here, heading northwest onto Hidden Cove Trail.

Continue down through a shady oak-dominated forest. After 0.2 miles from the end of Morena Butte Trail, the lake comes into view again and another 0.4 miles takes you to the gated end of the trail, where you can enjoy views of Lake Morena.

Heading back up Hidden Cove Trail, watch for a single-track path on your right. You might not have noticed it as you passed by the first time. But after backtracking about 0.4 miles, you'll discover the path in a washed-out area in a narrow meadow break in the trees.

This narrow path, the Hauser Overlook Trail, heads uphill but is not strenuous. Giving you a bird's-eye view of the surrounding area, the trail invites you to pause and look out over the lake, which reflects the sky—changing from blue to gray according to the weather. Watch, and listen, for rattlesnakes, especially in spring.

The trail continues up, bending to the west, where it ends on a rock cliff looking out to the west and down over the dam.

Standing on the edge of the cliff, ponder the history of Lake Morena, which includes a 1916 contract between a drought-riddled city of San Diego and Charles Hatfield, a man known as "the rainmaker." Shortly after Hatfield set up his towers near the dam and concocted his secret rain recipe that caused smoke to billow into the air . . . the rain began. It poured for days, deluging San Diego with so much rain that bridges washed away and homes slid off their foundations. Citizens then sued the city for damage to their property! The city never paid Hatfield, reasoning that the rain was an act of God rather than a result of Hatfield's magic.

Retrace your steps downhill to the main trail. When you reach the connecting section, turn right and follow it back to Ward's Flat Trail, which will deliver you to your car.

■ MORE FUN

The Campo Stone Store and Museum at 31130 CA 94 is an interesting historical diversion about 20 minutes from Lake Morena; call (619) 478-5707 for more information.

■ TO THE TRAILHEAD

From I-8 East, exit and turn right onto Buckman Springs Road, continuing west for about 6 miles. Turn right on Oak Drive and travel for another 1.5 miles to Lake Morena Drive. Turn right and drive straight into Lake Morena Regional Park. Pay for parking at the ranger booth, then continue just past a gate on the left (the trailhead), where you'll turn into a small dirt parking area.

■ OVERVIEW

LENGTH: 4.85 miles round-trip	parking area; portable toilets at frequent intervals around the lake
CONFIGURATION: Loop	
SCENERY: Native plants, shimmering water	**SPECIAL COMMENTS:** The best days to hike are Wednesday through Friday, when the loop is closed to automobiles. Picnic benches, barbecues, boating, and fishing make this a popular place, especially on weekends. Be prepared for company at any time; exercisers love the reservoir loop for jogging, inline skating, and biking. Obey the posted stay-to-the-right, pass-on-left signs for your safety. Leashed dogs allowed, but not within 50 feet of the water.
EXPOSURE: Open to sunlight	
TRAFFIC: Moderate–heavy	
TRAIL SURFACE: Asphalt paving	
HIKING TIME: 1.5–2 hours	
ACCESS: Free; open daily, sunrise–sunset	
MAPS: Available at www.sandiego.gov/water/recreation/miramar.shtml	
FACILITIES: Public restrooms near	

■ SNAPSHOT

This easy paved loop, framed by a verdant setting, is an excellent example of natural-resources management that makes a positive impact on the community. The tranquil eastern end fosters reflection and serenity, then slowly delivers visitors to the more urban western edges and a slow return to everyday life.

■ CLOSE-UP

In your car, bear right past the boat-launching area into the large south parking area. Begin at the kiosk, which features Project Wildlife information, near the public restrooms. With the reservoir on your left, head east. The paved road is quickly framed by native plants. Bushy lemonadeberry and chamise contrast with the more delicate leaves of twining wild-cucumber vines and the bright-red and coral blooms of monkey

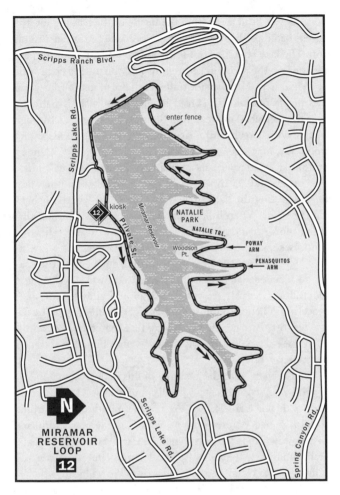

MIRAMAR
RESERVOIR
LOOP
12

flower. You'll also spot some nonnative vegetation. Eucalyptus trees, though common to and thriving in San Diego's climate, aren't indigenous. A few pines also mix into the landscape, as does cottony-plumed pampas grass.

As you head away from the bustle of the parking lot, the paved road dips slightly and a more peaceful setting surrounds you. The lake stretches out in fingerlike folds to your left, tall reeds lining the shore in some spots and the water's edge wide open in others. Narrow side trails reach down to the lake. Couples picnic on colorful spread blankets, and fishers patiently wait for a catch. The reservoir is stocked December through March with largemouth bass, bluegill, catfish, sunfish, and trout. You may also spot people fishing from boats. Canoes, motorboats, and rowboats are available for rent on weekends.

At about 0.75 miles, you'll round the lake's southeastern finger and spot the dam to the west, across the length of shimmering water. When full, Miramar Reservoir has a surface that spans more than 162 surface acres—dramatically reflecting sunrises, sunsets, and San Diego's beautiful skies.

The loop continues along this rural, quiet end of the lake, where hikers are occasionally interrupted by skate, bike, and foot traffic. Greet others with a smile or nod, allowing the lake's peaceful ambience to infuse you with goodwill returned by fellow visitors. Perhaps they're happy that the complete loop is open these days: crossing the dam was prohibited for about six years after 9-11.

In keeping with the anatomy of this body of water and its fingerlike points, at 2.5 miles you'll come to marked Penasquitos Arm, with side trails leading up into the hillsides. Just 0.1 mile ahead is signed Woodson Point, with a fishing pier and picnic area. Poway Arm is the next signed area, with an entry to Natalie Trail within a few steps. The optional narrow (but easy) side trail delivers you to Natalie Park, 3 miles from the trailhead, which is a lovely spot to picnic or simply rest in tree shade.

At 4 miles, you'll enter the chain-link fence–secured portion of the loop, which delivers you across the dam itself. Here, you'll begin to encounter slower foot traffic. Many people park in the small west lot at the lake and enjoy a stroll only along the dam. Others walk from neighboring communities, making views of the water the high point of their exercise routines without adding the entire loop. In any event, exit the fence-framed dam and head left, making the loop back toward the kiosk and your beginning point. You'll have walked 4.85 miles.

■ MORE FUN

Finish off your urban getaway with a taste of fine French cuisine. Escargot, shrimp, and vegetarian entrees await you at La Bastide Bistro, 10006 Scripps Ranch Boulevard, #104, just half a mile from Miramar Reservoir. Phone (858) 577-0033.

■ TO THE TRAILHEAD

From I-15, exit east on Mira Mesa Boulevard and travel 0.3 miles, then turn right on Scripps Ranch Boulevard. Travel 0.3 miles, then turn left on Scripps Lake Drive. The reservoir entrance is on the left, at 0.4 miles.

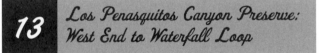

13 *Los Penasquitos Canyon Preserve:*
West End to Waterfall Loop

■ OVERVIEW

LENGTH: 6 miles

CONFIGURATION: Loop

SCENERY: Oak forest, birds, creek, and waterfall

EXPOSURE: Mostly sunny

TRAFFIC: Heavy on weekends

TRAIL SURFACE: Packed dirt, river rock, silt, and leaf litter

HIKING TIME: 3 hours

ACCESS: Free

MAPS: Available online at www.san diego.gov/park-and-recreation/parks/penasq.shtml

FACILITIES: Portable toilet at the West End parking lot

SPECIAL COMMENTS: Open from 8 a.m.–dusk. A favorite of many, the preserve sees numerous bicyclists, runners, and walkers on weekends. If you want a quiet hike, come on a weekday.

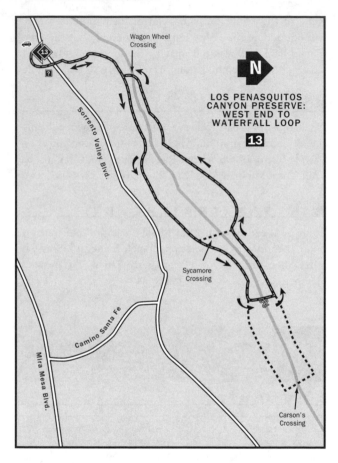

■ SNAPSHOT

The creek provides a relaxing riparian backdrop in this popular preserve. The 3,720-acre oasis of nature amid the traffic and city excitement offers a home to wildlife such as coyotes, birds, and rabbits.

■ CLOSE-UP

Access the trail at the east end of the large parking lot to head through the dense, cool shade provided by sycamore trees. At the kiosk about 100 yards from the trailhead, go left beneath the Sorrento Valley Boulevard bridge. Begin heading northeast, up the hill. The trail soon levels off.

In the spring, you'll spot fuzzy caterpillars also hiking this route. As if racing against the clock, the tiny creatures move quickly, leaving behind smooth channels in the dirt. On a recent visit, we counted 92. Look carefully. Perhaps you'll count even more.

The route descends into the canyon and joins another trail at about 0.6 miles. You'll head right (east) here and soon spot a sign marked "Wagon Wheel Crossing" on the left. Continue past this for now, taking note of the water level. Decide whether you will feel comfortable crossing from the other side or will need to find another route across the creek (other options are described below).

The route surface changes to coarse gravel and small, smooth river rocks as you continue east. Watch for bright red splashes of California fuchsia and perhaps see coyote scat full of fur—evidence of a thriving canyon population sustained by rabbits and other rodents. In the spring, you may hear pups practicing their yelps from within the off-trail brush, even during the day.

At 1.5 miles, a rocky viewpoint where the trail bends south offers a look up the creek toward the waterfall. The route straightens again, heading into oak forest with lots of shade. Wood roses are among the flowers here. You might also spot the feathery herb chamomile growing in clumps midtrail. Where there are flowers there are butterflies, and you'll likely see a variety flitting about here. Bigger river rocks make it easier to carefully cross this stretch.

At about 2 miles, you'll pass the "Sycamore Crossing" path on the left. Check the water level here to help you decide where to cross the creek. To reach the waterfall, continue another 1 mile east on mostly level ground that is open to the sunlight. Rocky in areas, the trail has a variety of sage and mint plants growing alongside it, pleasantly scenting the air. At the waterfall on the left, rock steps lead toward the water. On weekends you'll find bustling activity up and down the creek banks all around the waterfall. Some hikers choose to cross here, scampering across the rocks like agile mountain goats. Others meander upstream, then remove shoes to trek across the shallow waters. You could also continue on the main trail for about another 0.5 miles to Carson's Crossing, where there is a bridge, or stop here and return on the same route by which you came. Be wary of snakes that also visit this area. Rattlesnakes are not uncommon anywhere in the canyon, but are as attracted to the water as human visitors.

Assuming you've crossed near the waterfall, watch for poison oak as you head right and up the trail along the split-rail fencing. Head slightly east above the creek, then north back to a wide main trail, where you'll go left (west) to begin the return loop. After several yards, the trail splits right and left. Head left down toward the creek, where you get good views of the babbling water as it moves west.

Cross two cement bridges and continue on a path above the creek. The narrow path gradually loses altitude, descending almost to creek level for a time. Sycamores dot the meadow as the trail heads into open space and continues west. The canyon is quieter on this side of the creek. Watch and listen for signs of life: lizards, birds, and perhaps a cottontail rabbit hopping along in early morning or late afternoon looking for a snack. Be respectful of any wildlife and plants in the canyon. You'll notice multiple bicycle tire and foot tracks layered along the trail, where visitors do the least damage to this natural habitat. But having planned paths doesn't protect all the wildlife. Occasionally, a creature as fascinating as the seldom-seen millipede lies dead in the middle of the path—the victim of a fast-moving bicyclist.

If you decided on the way out that Sycamore Crossing is your best way across, watch for the sign about 1 mile from the waterfall. Cross, then take the trail on the south side of the creek back to the beginning. If you decided on Wagon Wheel Crossing, head left at the sign and wade through the water, or find a nearby shallower spot to get to the other side.

Once across, head west for a short distance, then south up over the hill. Under the bridge, the mule-fat bushes release cottony fuzz in the spring, spilling white bits of fluff into the air where they drift on the breeze. At the kiosk, head right and back to the parking lot and civilization.

■ TO THE TRAILHEAD

Take I-5 to Carmel Valley Road and drive east for 0.2 miles. At El Camino Real, turn right and continue for another mile to Carmel Mountain Road. Turn right, travel 0.6 miles to Sorrento Valley Road and turn left. Another 0.3 miles brings you to Sorrento Valley Boulevard. Turn left again (at the traffic signal) and go 1 mile to the staging area on the right.

14 Del Dios Gorge Trail

■ OVERVIEW

LENGTH: 2.2 miles round-trip

CONFIGURATION: Out-and-back

SCENERY: Views of water, chaparral

EXPOSURE: Open to sun

TRAFFIC: Light

TRAIL SURFACE: Silty soil

HIKING TIME: 0.75 hours

ACCESS: Free

MAPS: PDF downloadable at www.sdrp .org/archive/Trail%20Maps/Santa%20 Fe%20Valley-Del%20Dios%20Gorge %20(map%20side)%20FINAL.pdf

FACILITIES: None

SPECIAL COMMENTS: This wide, easy path is well-maintained and leads to the 180-foot Del Dios Gorge truss-style bridge. The trail is part of the Coast to Crest system of trails, which when finished, will stretch from the sea inland for more than 50 miles.

■ SNAPSHOT

Listen for the twanging call of red-winged blackbirds that inhabit the San Dieguito River. Some water is usually present close to the parking area, and increases as you near the bridge on this meandering multiuse trail suitable for beginners and a favorite of hikers with dogs.

■ CLOSE-UP

Head uphill on the paved route (west) toward the gate you see at the top of the hill (an alternative entry to The Crosby residential community). Del Dios Gorge Trail entry (marked) is on the left. You'll also spot the entry to the Santa Fe Valley Trail on the right. Although still closed as of this writing for bridge rebuilding due to the 2007 wildfires, check back for the Santa Fe Valley Trail's reopening soon. Its 3.72 round-trip miles travel through mixed rocky and flat terrain with views of the surrounding valley, and are worth a look.

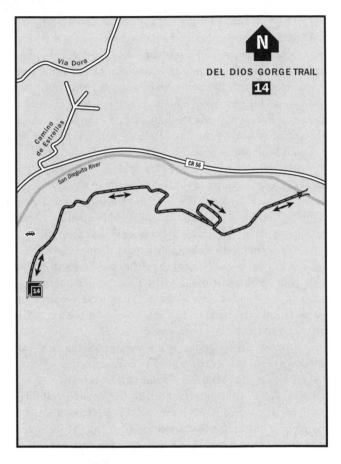

For now, head up the very gradual northerly grade of the Del Dios Gorge Trail, past a panel explaining about wildfires and how the land regenerates. You'll see evidence of the 2007 wildfires here in charred stalks sticking upright from the otherwise bushy greenery of lemonadeberry, which is recovering nicely.

The path bends to the left, and settles into a nearly flat walk heading east. In spring, the spiky paddles of the prickly-pear cactus erupt in sunrise-pink blooms that appear to glow. Another thorny plant grows in abundance here: thistle, with purple blooms that dry as the year wears on, and eventually rustle in fall breezes. You'll note the creamy spring blooms of California buckwheat, and the butterscotch-orange of California's golden poppies. Even an occasional mariposa lily pops its pale-pink flower head from the dry brush.

At approximately 0.4 miles, the trail jogs to the right and then back again a couple of times, and heads up slightly steeper slopes. In the hills across the Del Dios Highway, which is on your left, you'll see the remnants of an old aqueduct system held up on trellis platforms—a reminder of days gone by.

At just under 0.8 miles, pole fencing defines the narrowing trail that turns suddenly to the right heading south off the wide path (which continues east). Pass the bat information panel that expounds on the benefits of these wild creatures that eat pests and get a bad rap as being spooky. At the top of the hill, you'll go left—east again—down the hill.

Reach the truss bridge at 1.1 mile. Enjoy the view east and down to the reedy depths below. On clear days, the sky cuts a warm-blue swath into the surrounding hills as frame.

As of this writing (June 2009), the trail beyond the bridge is still under construction, so this is the stopping point. Upon completion, the trail will stretch clear to Lake Hodges and beyond. For now, linger above the water until, refreshed and renewed from your time in nature, you retrace your steps back to the starting point.

■ MORE FUN

Cielo Village just across the Del Dios Highway is a new retail area that might hold some interest. As with many new retail plazas, some flux has occurred with occupants. Otherwise, head east or west the way you came, back to the populated areas that hold your favorite eateries and pastimes.

■ TO THE TRAILHEAD

From I-5, take the Via de la Valle exit and head east approximately 7.5 miles. Turn right at an unmarked entry road across from the Cielo development. From I-15, exit at Via Rancho Parkway, drive west just less than 4 miles to Del Dios Highway, and turn left; then continue approximately 5 miles. Turn left just prior to the Cielo development (which is on the right). Or, take West Valley Parkway (west) which becomes Del Dios Highway after approximately 2 miles. Continue another 5 miles and turn left. The staging area is several hundred yards forward on the right.

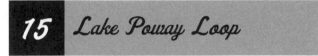

15 Lake Poway Loop

■ OVERVIEW

LENGTH: 2.6 miles

CONFIGURATION: Loop

SCENERY: Lake and waterfowl, picturesque views of boats atop the glistening water, chaparral, wildflowers

EXPOSURE: Open to sunlight

TRAFFIC: Moderately heavy

TRAIL SURFACE: Well-packed dirt, some areas of slippery loose dirt

HIKING TIME: 1.5 hours

ACCESS: Parking always free to Poway residents, and free to visitors November–March; April–October, weekends, and holidays, non-Poway residents pay a parking fee: $5 for auto, RV, bus, or $2 for motorcycle.

MAPS: Available from the city of Poway online at www.ci.poway.ca.us/lake_poway/index.html

FACILITIES: Public restrooms near parking lot; chemical toilets along the trail

SPECIAL COMMENTS: Open 7 a.m.– sunset. The trails are shared by equestrians and bicycle riders. Children under 10 may need a hand on the few steeper areas, especially in summer when the dry soil is loose. Call (858) 668-4770 for more information.

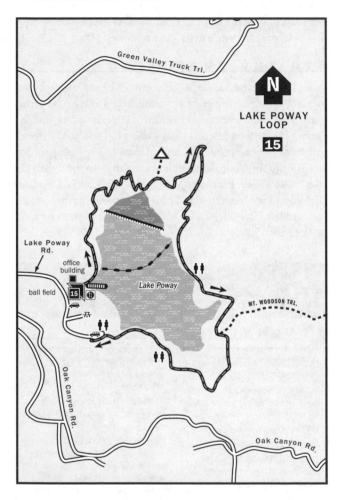

■ SNAPSHOT

The Lake Poway Recreation Area offers boat rentals and fishing, a walk-in campground, and a grassy picnic area. For day

hikers, even busy weekends in this spacious area let you feel close to nature and far from the city.

■ CLOSE-UP

A sense of pride pervades the city of Poway and spills over into its countryside and public recreation areas. With its pristine picnic areas and lake views reminiscent of a European vacation spot, hikers can immerse themselves in the relaxation of a long holiday, if only for an hour or two.

From the parking area, walk north past the office building on the left and look for the trail entrance to the left of the snack bar. You'll head north for several yards and get a view of the boat dock and the lake on your right, to the east. The wide trail, flanked by smallish pine trees that smell like Christmas all year, bends west and leads up a short, steep section before gradually descending northwest. Look for skullcap with purple blooms in spring and summer and wild cucumber and curly dock—all growing among sparse laurel sumac and sage scrub, which are regenerating since the 2007 wildfires. Since those fires, this already spring bloom–heavy lake loop is all but carpeted with flowers. Zillions of golden poppies intersperse with spring's rich color palette. Watch for fleabane (a natural flea repellent); its lavender daisies with yellow centers grow on spindly stems. Blue dicks—a member of the lily family—bloom as early as January, with showy yet delicate clusters that sway atop one- to two-foot, grasslike stems.

At about 0.5 miles, the trail gets steeper and a series of short switchbacks lead you down to the base of the dam. Smaller children might need a helping hand here, especially in dry months when loose ground gets slippery. Look to the northwest for a triangle of rocks peeking between the hills. It's the dam for Lake Ramona, about 4 miles away. When you get to the bottom of the downhill slope, you'll see a water trough for horses, and perhaps a few dragonflies hovering nearby. A creek runs here at the base of the dam, too, and you'll likely notice the creamy yellow flowers of Hooker's evening primrose during spring and summer. The festive blooms that grow on hairy stalks may be "dressed to kill," but the name doesn't refer to anything tawdry. They were named for a 19-century botanist. At about 1 mile from the trailhead, a path on the left leads off to the campground area, which is still closed as of this writing due to losses during the 2007 Witch Creek Fire.

The trail continues to the right, climbing gradually upward from the dam. At about 1.5 miles, you'll start to see the dam again. A little farther and the lake is back in view as the trail gradually descends. On weekends, the glistening water is dotted with picturesque rowboats, and you make your way down to the water. You'll likely hear laughter drifting across the lake from the picnic park near your car. As you get closer to the water, you'll hear the clicking and squabbling of the American coot, which gathers in groups on the lake. My family has nicknamed this ever-present bird the American "toot," because its voice is so similar to a child's bicycle horn.

As the trail levels out, you'll see portable toilets. A short path leads down to a beaching area for boats. Pine trees used to shade this area, making it a comfortable resting spot to sit and watch the water lap at the shore. In fact, several yards forward a shaded lake overlook bench was marked "Pine Point." It is unclear yet whether or how this favorite picnic spot will be recreated.

The trail meanders around the northernmost inlet, then comes to a fork. Keep heading to the right around the lake and bypass the Mount Woodson Trail opening to the left. You'll start to climb again, but at just more than 2 miles, the trail slopes downward and heads past a side trail that leads to the lake's southern shore and the boat dock. Take this trail if you choose, or head up the trail, at times lined with milk thistle. The spiny plants sprout purple blooms in the summer. When you reach the picnic park, head across the grassy knolls to your car. In the spring, my daughters like to pluck the clover blooms that grow profusely in the lawn, tying them together for a natural chain that brings back childhood memories for me. Press the chains into a book to hold onto the memory of a pleasant day at Lake Poway.

■ MORE FUN

Old Poway Park is a historical gem with a museum, an operating steam train, and a Saturday farmer's market. From Lake Poway, turn left onto Espola Road. Drive just over 3 miles to Twin Peaks and turn right. At about 0.8 miles, turn left on Midland. The 4.75-acre park is about 0.5 miles on the right at 14134 Midland Road. Call (858) 679-4313 for more information.

■ TO THE TRAILHEAD

From I-15, take Rancho Bernardo Road and head east. Rancho Bernardo Road becomes Espola Road after about 2 miles. Travel a total of just under 5 miles and turn left on Lake Poway Road. Proceed to the entrance booth and park in the lot.

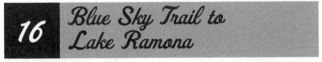

16 Blue Sky Trail to Lake Ramona

■ OVERVIEW

LENGTH: 4.5 miles

CONFIGURATION: Out-and-back

SCENERY: Views of Lake Ramona, distant Lake Poway, birds, creek lined with sycamores, oak forest, and a variety of flowering plants along the upper trail

EXPOSURE: Shady with some dappled sunlight on entry trail; full sun on trail to lake

TRAFFIC: Heavy

TRAIL SURFACE: Packed dirt, leaf litter on creekside trail

HIKING TIME: 2.5 hours

ACCESS: Free

MAPS: Free at kiosk beyond trailhead; also viewable at www.blueskyreserve.org

FACILITIES: Portable toilets near entry, in picnic area, and above Lake Ramona

SPECIAL COMMENTS: Leashed dogs are permitted (on main trail only, not the creekside trail). No bicycles or motor vehicles are allowed. Horses permitted on the main trail only—not on the streamside trail. For recorded information, phone (858) 668-4781.

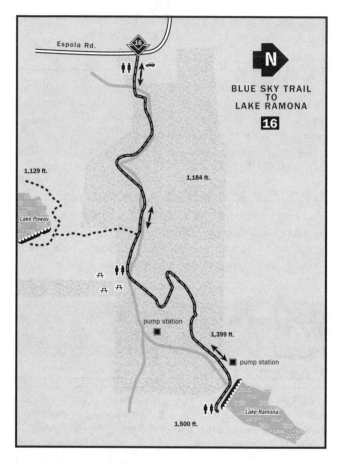

■ SNAPSHOT

Oak woodland, riparian habitat, coastal sage scrub, and chaparral lend variety to this oasis near the suburbs of Poway. The first 1.5-mile stretch is a flat walk through dappled shade in woodland recovering from fire, which makes the Lake Ramona Trail fork a logical turnaround point for anyone not wanting an uphill hike.

■ CLOSE-UP

Park in the lot and head south along the street for a few yards before turning to the left (east) down the dirt road that begins this trail. Very close to the trailhead, old oaks that once allowed only small patches for a view of the sky—and made one wonder about the reserve's name—are now recovering from fire, so give off less shade. On this nice flat stretch, enjoy the stately oaks' regenerative powers as they more fully recover from the fires over time.

At approximately 0.25 miles, you'll notice the "Oak Grove" marker sign for a narrow trail descending on the left side of the wide main trail. Take the side trail down toward the creek that runs along the north side of the trail. You will see an ancient grove of oaks to the left. Sunlight filters through the canopy in glints of gold, producing a hazy, enchanted atmosphere. Baby oaks stand like spindly weeds, while their towering parent trees reach with outstretched limbs as if gathering the seedlings under protective wings. Be careful to stay on the trail to avoid trampling the young oaks. You'll note the 2007 fire's devastation, which has thinned the canopy, but the enchantment remains.

Listen to the frogs' chorus rising from underlayer of fallen leaves and limbs tangled with the vines of wild roses and poison oak. Alongside the narrow trail strewn with acorns and decaying oak leaves, clusters of fat toadstools sprout from a fluffy orange carpet of leaves, dropped in the fall by the western sycamores growing immediately adjacent to the stream. Look for toadstools on the other side of the trail, too. A variety of them grow here in the cool forest shade. Flattened and with fluted edges, or round as buttons, or shaped like a beanie cap, they burst from the ground, making the moist dirt clumps form a tiny earthen fence around the fleshy stems.

At approximately half a mile from the hike's start, the 0.3-mile streamside trail reconnects with the broader main route, where horses are allowed. Pass the side trail, marked Lake Poway, off to the right. Another 0.2 miles brings you to an area that, prior to the fires, held picnic tables—which have not yet been replaced at the time of this writing. You've come 1.1 mile from your car. When you reach the sign pointing left to Lake Ramona, turn left. (The main trail leads to a water tower and pump station, and beyond that a private residence—none of which are public areas.)

After turning left at the Lake Ramona fork, emerge into sunlight. Bring drinking water, even in moderate spring and fall weather. You'll hear the roar of the pump station, which comes into view as the trail begins its gradual, 400- to 500-foot ascent to Lake Ramona to the northeast. The trail gets steeper for a short distance, switching back to the west. Don't let the somewhat barren, wide dirt trail fool you into thinking this will be a dull hike. As the path switches back, climbing steadily and gradually to the east, surprisingly delightful foliage awaits. Blooming with tiny white flowers well into autumn, wild cucumber twines up into the branches of laurel sumac growing along the trail. Bright-orange clumps of parasitic California dodder, more commonly called "witch's hair," winds around both the cucumber and the laurel sumac. The knotty orange tangles thrive at lower elevations, disappearing as the trail climbs higher. Lupine and a variety of mint begin to appear in bushy tufts along the inner edge of the trail, resting against the rocky face where the road has been cut into the mountain. This hiking route is actually the old Green Valley Truck Trail but is no longer open to motor traffic.

At just shy of 2 miles, asphalt replaces the dirt road. Getting closer to the lake, a wall of rock rises ahead to the east. Here, closer to the water, tree tobacco grows. Its narrow yellow flowers seem to drip from the ends of spindly stalks. The road becomes asphalt where Blue Sky Ecological Reserve land ends and the Ramona Water District begins. Pause and look to the southwest, where the trail etches down the mountain. Lake Poway, about 2 miles away, sparkles in the sunlight. Turkey vultures circle overhead, giving parents an opportunity to tease any children who are tuckered out from the hike—maybe those vultures are circling above a weary hiker who collapsed! You will pass another pump station on the left before the asphalt road bends to the south. Avocado groves growing above the road come into view and, as you reach the top, the plumed branches of commercially grown palms line the hillsides to the southeast.

To work out a different set of muscles, or just for fun, walk backward on this last, smooth stretch of asphalt. Once at the top, enjoy a view over the vast blue waters of Lake Ramona from the guardrail. You'll have come 2.25 miles. The dense quietude is interrupted only by the quack and flutter of ducks gathered near the lake's shore, or by an occasional small airplane heading east to the airstrip in Ramona.

The trip back down feels entirely different than the climb, which can be tiring, especially in warmer weather. But passing breezes will cool your damp shirt as you make your way back down with the help of gravity. My family likes to stop at the picnic area on the way out of the reserve, eating the lunch we pack for the trip.

■ MORE FUN

A treat for both the eyes and the taste buds can be found at the Hamburger Factory Restaurant. Old-fashioned memorabilia, a friendly neighborhood atmosphere, and an inexpensive menu that includes barbecued chicken, ribs, and much more than the name implies offer diners an experience sure to satisfy. From Blue Sky Ecological Reserve, turn left onto Espola Road. Drive for approximately 3 miles and turn right on Twin Peaks. At about 0.8 miles, turn left on Midland. The restaurant is about 0.5 miles down on the right at 14122 Midland Road, Poway. Call (858) 486-4575.

■ TO THE TRAILHEAD

From I-15, exit at Rancho Bernardo Road and travel east for 3.5 miles. Note that the road becomes Espola Road at the Summerfield intersection. Watch for the Blue Sky Ecological Reserve sign on the left, and turn into the nearby parking lot. The trailhead is to the right.

■ OVERVIEW

LENGTH: 4.5 miles	**MAPS:** Call (858) 674-2270
CONFIGURATION: One-way	**FACILITIES:** There is a portable toilet
SCENERY: Views of the lake, birds, and	across the street from trailhead, rest-
a creek	rooms near the concession stand, and
EXPOSURE: Mostly sunny	another portable toilet along the lake.
TRAFFIC: Heavy on weekends	**SPECIAL COMMENTS:** During fishing
TRAIL SURFACE: Sandy dirt	season, a concession stand is open
HIKING TIME: 3.5 hours	near the picnic area.
ACCESS: Free	

■ SNAPSHOT

This easy hike is overrun by bicyclists on the weekends, but weekdays (outside fishing season) are quiet and serene.

■ CLOSE-UP

From the parking lot, head south on the paved walkway that makes the first section accessible for people with disabilities. I-15 runs along the right side of this paved area for about 0.5 miles. Sage scrub, black sage, and California buckwheat grow close to the trail, scenting the air. On windy days, the rustling of grasses in the meadows to the left sounds like ocean waves and dulls the roar of traffic on the adjacent interstate.

The walkway bends to the right, ducking under the freeway. In the spring, cliff swallows gather by the thousands, swooping to and from their mud nests beneath the freeway. The paved walkway bears right in the cool shade where cyclists speed by (be careful!) and heads north for a short distance until the pavement ends and the dirt trail begins.

Turn left onto the level trail to head southwest. Notice that old cracked asphalt clings to the ground in some places,

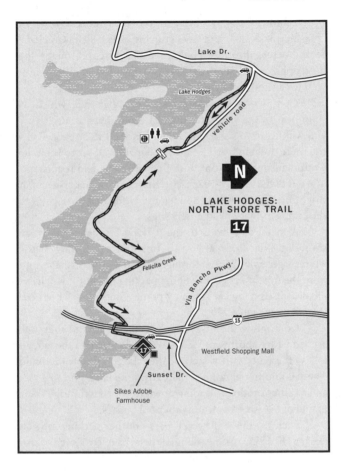

Lake Dr.

Lake Hodges

vehicle road

N

LAKE HODGES:
NORTH SHORE TRAIL

17

Felicita Creek

Via Rancho Pkwy.

15

17

Westfield Shopping Mall

Sunset Dr.

Sikes Adobe
Farmhouse

remnants of Old Highway (US) 395, which served as the main
vehicle road until the interstate was built.

The route bends to the right, heading northwest, and the
freeway sounds begin to fade, leaving the airwaves open to
birdsong. Quails, startled from their foraging in the brush, will
flutter across the path, and finches twitter in the bush.

Another 0.25 miles bring the trail to an oasis of sorts, with sprawling oaks and palm trees growing near Felicita Creek. Use rocks to cross the creek (bicyclists splash right through), then head uphill about 50 yards. The trail turns left, climbing southwest for a short distance.

Continue southwest on the wide, flat trail, which will soon bear to the right (northwest) again. Even in drier years, you will begin to see the lake water along this stretch. Follow the route downhill; a 0.5-mile stretch runs closer to the water. Cottontails may dart out onto the path here, and roadrunners hop out of the prickly-pear cactus that grows in massive clumps. Bright-orange California dodder and wild cucumber vines top the cactus formations like zany wigs.

A metal gate leads to the parking lot, concessions, and restrooms—facilities are open only during fishing season, which is generally March through October. The hike continues from the northwest corner of the parking lot, but if you like to picnic, this is a logical stopping point. Grassy areas hold tree-shaded picnic tables.

Continuing the hike, you will turn right and follow the asphalt path a short way. Watch for the dirt trail on the left, and follow the path with a view of the lake for about 0.25 miles. There is another parking lot here; this one has a portable toilet and a cement pathway leading down to the lake through stands of mulefat, leather root, and other tall bushes.

Back on the trail, you'll pass another parking area and reach a shady area and parking lot near Lake Drive across from the Del Dios Country Store.

■ MORE FUN

Back at the Sunset Drive trailhead, you can cross the road to see the Sikes Adobe Farmhouse that was built from adobe bricks in the late 1800s and is one of the oldest structures in San Diego County.

■ TO THE TRAILHEAD

To do this as a one-way hike, take cars on I-15 to Via Rancho Parkway and head west for 3 miles. Turn left on Lake Drive and park across from Del Dios Country Store, about 0.9 miles from the Lake Drive turnoff. In the second vehicle, travel back up to Via Rancho Parkway and head east for about 3.5 miles. Turn right on Sunset Drive and follow it less than 0.1 mile to the end, where there is a small parking lot at the trailhead.

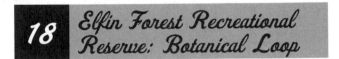

18 *Elfin Forest Recreational Reserve: Botanical Loop*

■ OVERVIEW

LENGTH: 1.5 miles

CONFIGURATION: Loop (balloon with string)

SCENERY: Native plants, described with interesting facts in the "Botanical Trail Guide," available in box at the trail's start, or online at www .olivenhain.com/trail_map.html

EXPOSURE: Sunny and shady

TRAFFIC: Moderate

TRAIL SURFACE: Earthen path, leaf litter

HIKING TIME: 30 minutes

ACCESS: Free

MAPS: Available at kiosk near parking area, or online at www.olivenhain .com/trail_map.html

FACILITIES: Restrooms near parking area

SPECIAL COMMENTS: The reserve is open 8 a.m. to 45 minutes before sunset every day except Christmas. The Botanical Loop is designated hiking only and includes a creek crossing. For more information about the reserve, call (760) 753-6466, ext. 147.

■ SNAPSHOT

This well-maintained trail offers a quiet, easy loop that makes it perfect for any age. The "Botanical Trail Guide" published by reserve staff lends an educational element that makes this foray into nature even richer.

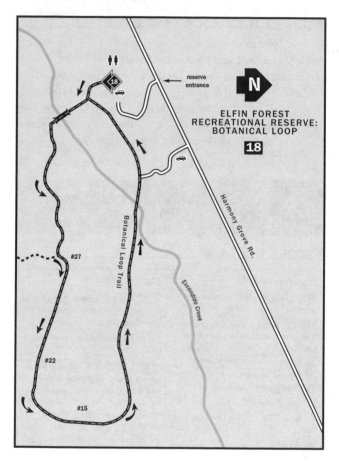

■ CLOSE-UP

To access the Botanical Loop Trail, head south across the cement creek bridge as if to hike the Way Up Trail, which is marked by a sign near the reserve's entrance. Once across the cement, turn right and walk uphill for about 200 feet. The trail bends east, connecting with the Botanical Loop Trail after about 0.5 miles.

Take a "Botanical Trail Guide" from the box on the left and head down the hill onto the loop trail. Numbered marker poles correspond with informative paragraphs in the guide. From this direction, begin with number 27, hollyleaf cherry, a bushy plant with hollylike leaves. Have you ever wondered about the reddish-brown fruit often seen hanging from small oak trees? No, they're not oak apples, oak oranges, or any other oak fruit. Number 22 identifies the ping-pong–sized balls as "galls" made when the California gall wasp lays its eggs in the stem. When the larvae emerge from their eggs, they release a chemical that causes the stem to swell into a gall. The gall provides food and protection for the tiny wasps.

Some plants aren't included in the guide, like the clumps of thistle, with their "milk"-splattered leaves, which grow on the right of the trail almost from the start of the loop. The tangy, herbaceous scent of black sage wafts up as the trail levels and heads east through the partial shade of oak trees.

Continuing, the route turns left (north), beginning the loop formation, and gradually descends at an easy grade. The ground is rocky here but not dangerously so. A bench in the shade awaits at number 15. Mountain mahogany is the featured plant here. This tree or shrub grows on the dry hillsides of San Diego County and provides shade for a variety of other plants.

Make the curve to the left and head west, moving into the denser shade of thicker oak forest. You'll hear the creek running, and within a few more steps, spot water gurgling over the large, flat rocks you'll use to cross. Heed the posted warnings. The creek crossing is a natural one and can be dangerous when the water is high. Use common sense and caution.

Once across, notice the arroyo willow, with its feathery blooms that turn to cottony fuzz. You'll see a road on the right that leads to a second parking lot. Pass this and continue west to the reserve's entrance. The path ahead, framed by placed rocks and pole-and-cable fencing, leads the way back to the marker for the Way Up Trail, the entrance, and your car.

■ TO THE TRAILHEAD

From I-15 South, take the Auto Parkway exit and turn left. Then turn left on Ninth Avenue, at the traffic signal. Proceed on Ninth, across the Valley Parkway intersection; the road bends sharply left. Ninth Avenue becomes Hale here. Continue on Hale to Harmony Grove Road. To stay on Harmony Grove you must make the first two left turns; otherwise, you'll end up on Enterprise or Kauana Loa. Past the second left turn, proceed on Harmony Grove Road to Elfin Forest Recreational Reserve, which appears on the left 1.5 miles past Country Club Drive. Turn left into the parking lot.

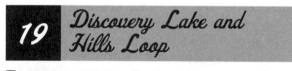

19 Discovery Lake and Hills Loop

■ OVERVIEW

LENGTH: 2.5 miles	www.ci.san-marcos.ca.us/departments.asp?id=2825
CONFIGURATION: Loop	
SCENERY: Waterfowl, lake, surrounding homes	**FACILITIES:** None
EXPOSURE: Sunny	**SPECIAL COMMENTS:** It can be quite hot on these trails that are mainly surrounded by blacktop streets in a newer neighborhood where vegetation isn't yet mature. Bring water and be prepared for lots of kids, joggers, and dog walkers around the lake itself—especially on weekends.
TRAFFIC: Moderate	
TRAIL SURFACE: Asphalt and soft soil	
HIKING TIME: 1 hour	
ACCESS: Free	
MAPS: Available at the trailhead kiosk at Lakeview Park, and online at	

■ SNAPSHOT

An urban trek that varies in appearance from park to greenbelt to open chaparral, this loop is used by locals as an exercise route. Local retirement centers bring seniors here to walk the

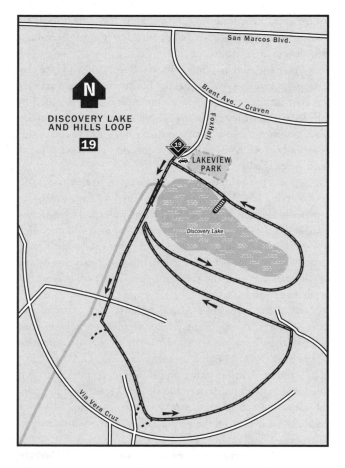

paved lake path, where they mingle with neighborhood families. The small lake holds a bevy of coots and ducks that gather at a dock for those who feed them.

■ CLOSE-UP

Follow the asphalt to the right of the parking lot for just a few steps to reach the lake. From the bridge, watch a heron or egret fishing, with their long legs and necks as the perfect tools for wading and dipping their beaks into the water—seemingly effortless in their habits.

Alive with ducks, coots, fish, and frogs, the small lake glistens in the sun. Despite the nearby houses and human activity, the animals appear at ease in an environment surrounded by tall reeds, where they can easily retreat. According to city of San Marcos information, bobcats and deer have also been spotted here. Early morning hours are probably best if you hope to see these more elusive creatures.

Across the bridge, you could continue on the paved lake path, curving left and looping around the lake for a short, 0.8-mile walk. For this longer trek, go right instead, on the downward sloping dirt trail past the bridge. The path will curve left toward nearby houses. Oak trees offer some shade on this section. A side trail leads off to the left, but you'll pass this by and continue along with the creek on your right; off-season, the creek may be dry.

At about 0.75 miles, you'll come to a paved road that heads into the housing complex. Be careful of cars as you cross a street, then hook up with a dirt path on the opposite side. Ignore that right fork that crosses the creek, and instead go uphill. Bushy chamise grows abundantly. Also notice straggly tree tobacco, with its smooth bluish-green leaves and cylindrical yellow-green blooms that may appear year-round. Its spindly limbs sway in even the gentlest of breezes—which may be all you get inland on hot days.

At a little over 1 mile, the trail splits off into the housing tract on the right. Take the left path uphill; do the same when the path splits again. These plentiful side routes make the paths convenient for nearby residents. Continue to the left, heading up the moderately steep hill that curves to follow the route of Via Vera Cruz, the vehicle road down below. Here, on the chaparral-covered hillside, the hike begins to feel more rural. After little more than a third of a mile, the path delivers you along the ridge with views to the east, beyond the quarry, and into the mountains. On clear days, you really can see forever—or close to it. Unfortunately, clear skies mean a view of brown smog as well, sometimes hanging like a dismal tent above the earth in the distance.

You'll pass houses very close on the right. Continue east, moving downhill with the view on the left and fenced backyards on the right. When you reach pavement again, head left to go back down the hill toward the lake. If you're feeling adventurous, hook up with the Double Peak Trail to the right. Leading about 1 mile to an elevation of 1,644 feet, Double Peak affords panoramic views of the Pacific Ocean to the west and mountains to the north and east. Assuming you've turned left, Discovery Lake comes back into view. The blue-green oasis contrasts sharply with the barren quarry's ugly rock-crushing machines hulking in the distance. When the quarry is silent, the tooting calls of coots squabbling on the water grow louder.

At the bottom, head right for a 0.8-mile trip around the lake before going back. The pleasant loop is lined with berry bushes and native plants (marked with signs), and the calls of the coots splashing on the lake fill the air. The ashen-colored birds splash noisily about, quarreling endlessly among themselves—but they're also very smart. According to a recent study by a University of California, Santa Cruz biologist that was published in the journal *Nature,* the birds can count and keep track of how many eggs they lay. Coots who don't win prime nesting spots don't give up their chance to have offspring either. They lay their eggs in other birds' nests—maybe that's what all the squabbling is about!

Where the lake loop bears left, making the curve around to the other side, you'll see a rickety-looking conveyer track and metal machinery sticking up against the open sky on the right (behind the chain-link fence). This is part of a rock quarry—quiet on weekends, the hulking stillness of the machinery adds a ghost-town feel to the surroundings.

■ MORE FUN

If you're hungry after your hike, turn left on San Marcos Boulevard and drive for about 1 mile to San Marcos's restaurant row. Cuisine runs the gamut from Thai to Mexican to seafood.

■ TO THE TRAILHEAD

Take CA 78 to San Marcos Boulevard and drive west for 0.5 miles to Bent Avenue, then turn left. Almost immediately, Bent becomes Craven. Drive 0.3 miles and turn right on Foxhall. Proceed another 0.2 miles and you'll run right into the parking area for Lakeview Park.

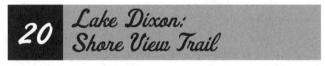

**20   Lake Dixon:
Shore View Trail**

■ OVERVIEW

LENGTH: 3 miles	**MAPS:** Free at the Ranger Station
CONFIGURATION: Out-and-back	**FACILITIES:** Public restrooms at the parking lot near picnic area; portable toilets along the trail
SCENERY: Lake, birds, chaparral, wildflowers	
EXPOSURE: Mostly sunny	**SPECIAL COMMENTS:** Open daily, 6 a.m.–sunset; weekends and weekdays are like night and day. For a peaceful commune with nature, hike this easy, family-friendly trail on non-holiday weekdays. As always when near water, be alert and supervise children.
TRAFFIC: Heavy on weekends; light on weekdays	
TRAIL SURFACE: Packed dirt	
HIKING TIME: 1.5 hours	
ACCESS: $3 parking fee on weekends and holidays; seniors age 60 and over free	

■ SNAPSHOT

There's something about ambling along a large body of water that calms the spirit. Unbelievably peaceful on weekdays, Dixon Lake is a slice of inland paradise: sage scrub, wildflowers, birds, and water all combine to make this an easy, rewarding hike.

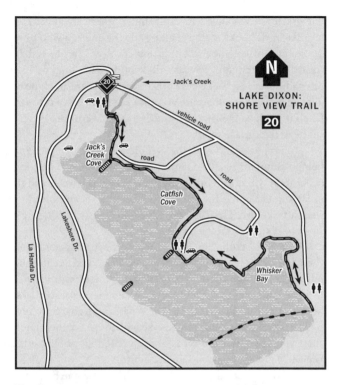

■ CLOSE-UP

From the parking area, proceed northeast and find the trail marker near the vehicle road. The rock-edged path heads south, just above the grassy picnic area, and continues a short distance past some small pines and acacias where scrub jays flutter. The trail gets a little rocky as it gradually descends, bringing the north-western edge of the lake into view. A wooden footbridge crosses Jack's Creek, which slows to a trickle in summer and fall.

Past the footbridge, the trail heads around the cattail-filled Jack's Creek Cove and bends to the left toward the pier. A breathtaking view of the entire lake stretches out to the east, making it feel as if you've stumbled into paradise. The brilliant blue-green water is alive with squabbling American coots. The duck like birds hunt for a meal alongside the anglers, who pose like statues in their boats. The lively coots are fun to watch. Tread lightly, though. The ash-dark birds with bright-white bills glide away in a V of gentle breakwater as you near. If you're quiet and catch one unaware, you may see a bird dive through the clear water to the lake bottom, grab a tasty crustacean, and paddle to the surface to eat.

You can walk out onto the first pier to see anglers hanging their poles out for a catch. Continuing on the trail, you will find lots of areas where you can easily get closer to the water and sit on large rocks along the shore. You'll find a second pier just past Catfish Cove. There is a portable toilet in the parking area, a few short steps from the trail.

The sage scrub thins and you'll come to a drier section where the trail is higher above the water. The coots like to hang out here, near Bass Cove, where they're hidden from view of the path. You'll hear them, though. With a series of short clicks, they warn of your presence; the birds pass the signal from one to the next. These sounds intersperse with longer, higher notes. Close your eyes and the birds' more excited squabbling may conjure the image of a child's bicycle horn.

Head on around to Whisker Bay, where people fish from the shore. When you reach the bench at a fork in the path, go right. You'll pass through a cool, shady area where ferns cascade down the decomposing granite alongside the trail, and willows and overgrown laurel sumac tangle with wild berry and wild cucumber vines. Sage and mint grow in abundance on this stretch as well, pleasantly scenting the air.

The trail widens into an open rock face approaching the buoy line, which marks the end of the hike. Dusky-brown cormorants balance on the cable line and atop the oblong red buoys, drying their not-quite-waterproof wings in the sun. With their long necks outstretched, they keep a cautious eye on anyone watching them. It's difficult to get a photograph of these ultrawary birds. They will fly away even as you aim your camera. Enjoy the cormorants for the time you can—they serve as a good reminder to enjoy every moment, a mentality that will serve you well while hiking.

As you head back, focus on the vegetation. Mesmerized by the water, you may have missed it on the way. From early spring through late summer, you will likely see skullcap, with its upright, dark-purple flowers. California fuchsia, sometimes called honeysuckle trumpet, blooms in profusion here. I've seen the narrow, orange-red flowers right into fall here at the lake. California lilac offers delicate clusters of pale blue–lilac flowers that contrast with the dark-green leaves of the shrub. When you reach the bench at the trail fork, you can turn right and head west up to the vehicle road. The trail ends here, where there are two portable toilets, and you can walk along the vehicle road if you choose.

■ TO THE TRAILHEAD

Take I-15 to the El Norte Parkway exit. Travel east on El Norte for about 4 miles to La Honda Drive, then turn left. Follow the road to the top, and turn right into the gate for Lake Dixon. Make an immediate right and park in the lot.

21 Los Jilgueros Preserve Trail

■ OVERVIEW

LENGTH: 1.5 miles

CONFIGURATION: Loop

SCENERY: Birds, stream, ponds, frogs, waterfowl, trees, and native plants

EXPOSURE: Some sunny and some shady

TRAFFIC: Moderately heavy

TRAIL SURFACE: Dirt and boardwalk

HIKING TIME: 45 minutes

ACCESS: Free

MAPS: None

SPECIAL COMMENTS: In this 46-acre preserve that is the most popular of the sites managed by the Fallbrook Land Conservancy, visitors find it easy to understand the necessity of preserves as cities grow and encroach on nature. Even with busy Mission Road to the west and a housing tract to the east, this space teems with animal and plant life, and offers a natural respite. Dogs on leashes are allowed—and common!

■ SNAPSHOT

A pleasant, 1.5-mile loop frames two ponds in this well-managed site that is popular with bikers, dog walkers, and those out for an invigorating walk through nature.

■ CLOSE-UP

Notice kiosks to the left of the parking lot and head into the preserve just past those. A bench placed at the start of the trail sets the tone for this adventure—easy-paced with lots of places to reflect.

After the short northwestern stretch that passes sycamore trees and scented sage, a wood-plank bridge appears on the left. Head across the bridge, where yerba mansa grows all around. The flowers' conical centers stretch up above white petals that form the crowning bloom for bright-green leaves on red stems. In winter, the plants die back to an ugly matte brown. This westward walk of a few hundred yards takes you closer to Mission Road, which runs along the outside of the preserve. The

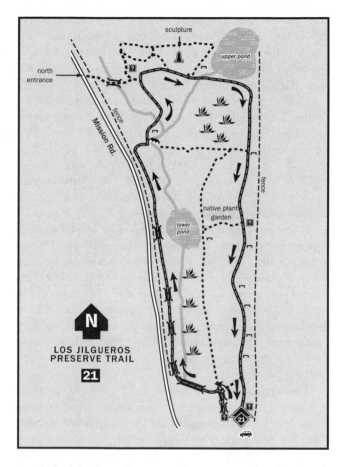

north
entrance

sculpture

upper pond

fence

Mission Rd.

native plant
garden

lower
pond

fence

N

**LOS JILGUEROS
PRESERVE TRAIL**

21

wood-plank bridge will cross water at some point; how much water depends on the season and rainfall amounts.

Where the plank bridge ends, turn right onto the dirt path. The route heads north alongside Mission Road for close to 0.5 miles, passing a series of short wood-plank bridges along the way. This stretch is considered the "nature trail." Dragonflies buzz, birds sing exuberantly, and cottontails hop in and out of the bushes. Thistles reach up, their purple blooms turning to tufts of fuzz as spring becomes summer. At two-thirds of the way in on the nature trail, notice the lower pond to your right. Vegetation makes the pond inaccessible. Stay on the path, respecting the area's designation as a preserve.

The trail bends to the right and continues. Look for another path on the left, heading northeast down into the trees. Take this route, where you'll see a concrete silt dam and a bench overlooking the creek. Here in the shade of the trees, you'll spot frogs lazing in the shallow creek water. Bright-orange nasturtiums thrive in this cool, shady environment where spotty sunlight filters down. Butterflies flit about and birdsong fills the air.

After spending time reflecting, cross the small bridge and head left into the open for a moment before reaching the shade of trees again. You'll notice another kiosk with information about the preserve up ahead. Two trails run off to the left of the kiosk. One crosses a wood-plank bridge toward the north entrance. The other, a single-track trail, delivers visitors up to the "firescape" garden, which is worth a look for those interested in native California plants that retard fire. If you choose to stroll through the garden, you can still access the main loop from that path later.

Sticking to the main loop trail, walk to the right up the hill (northeast). After a short distance, you will see the upper pond on the left. A short trail on the left leads to a bench near the shore that is shaded by lush pecan trees—a nice place to sit awhile and enjoy the birds. Continuing east on the path leads you along the right side of the pond.

The route turns abruptly southward for a long trek. Notice the rusty frame of an old truck and some old farm equipment partially hidden in the weeds on either side, remnants of the town of Fallbrook's history.

You'll come to a kiosk, and to the right of the path, see a native plant garden that blooms in a variety of colors in spring.

The showy Matilija poppy—which blooms in spring and summer—grows in the garden. The large, yellow-centered flowers with crinkly white petals have a uniquely pungent scent. A trail leads down around the garden (which may look bedraggled by summer) to a shaded bench near the lower pond.

The main loop trail continues south all the way back to the parking area. Benches along the way allow visitors to stop and reflect while enjoying birdsong and the sound of gentle winds.

■ MORE FUN

The Gem and Mineral Society Museum is nearby at 123 West Alvarado, across the street from Fallbrook's Art & Cultural Center. For more information, call (760) 728-1130. Air Park Road (almost directly across Mission from the preserve entrance) will take you to picnic benches that overlook Fallbrook Air Park, affording views of the afternoon's takeoffs and landings.

■ TO THE TRAILHEAD

Take I-15 North to the Pala/CA 76 exit and go left (west) 4.9 miles and turn right onto Mission Road. After 4.4 miles, you'll see signs for Los Jilgueros Preserve, which is past the high school and just past the Sterling Bridge intersection. Turn right and head down the dirt road, then park in the dirt- and bark-surfaced lot on the left.

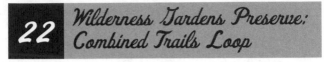

■ OVERVIEW

LENGTH: 3 miles

CONFIGURATION: Two connected loops with short out-and-back at end

SCENERY: Trees, pond, animal tracks, flowers, views of lower meadow and San Luis Rey River when the water is running

EXPOSURE: Mostly shady

TRAFFIC: Light

TRAIL SURFACE: Packed dirt

HIKING TIME: 2.5 hours

ACCESS: $2 self-pay parking fee

MAPS: Available at trailhead kiosk

FACILITIES: Chemical toilets at parking lot and on the trail

SPECIAL COMMENTS: Open Thursday–Monday, 8 a.m.–4 p.m.; closed Tuesday, Wednesday, and Christmas Day; closed during the entire month of August due to heat. No drinking water available. Pets are not permitted in the preserve. No horses, bicycles, or motor vehicles are allowed. Visitors under the age of 18 must be accompanied by an adult. For information, call (760) 742-1631. A recorded message gives current conditions, such as preserve closures due to rain or heat. Callers can leave a message to schedule a guided tour with the ranger.

■ SNAPSHOT

The pond, quiet forest, meadows, and hillside scenery make this preserve a relaxing retreat that doesn't require a long drive. Even on weekends, you may be the only hiker on these seldom-used trails.

■ CLOSE-UP

What's great about Wilderness Gardens Preserve is that there are several individual trails for hikers wanting to make a number of short visits. This description covers three trails that make a loop, giving you a 3-mile trek that enables you to see nearly everything the preserve has to offer.

Peaceful and tranquil best describe the 700-acre Wilderness Gardens Preserve in Pala. For thousands of years, this area was used only by Native Americans. The Upper Meadow Trail

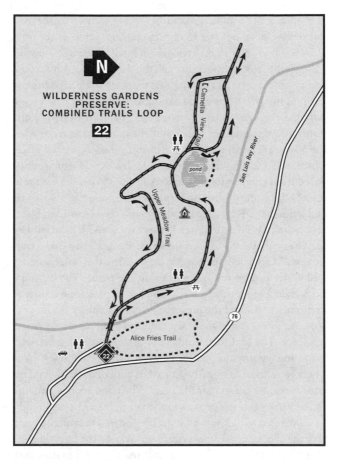

N

WILDERNESS GARDENS
PRESERVE:
COMBINED TRAILS LOOP

22

E Camellia View Trail

San Luis Rey River

pond

Upper Meadow Trail

Alice Fries Trail

76

22

seems untouched by modern civilization. And when walking along the narrow path, one can almost imagine going back to that very time.

To begin, head west from the parking area across the San Luis Rey riverbed, which, in California's drought conditions, is usually dry. A wooden footbridge was put here five years ago when heavy rains washed away the concrete. Except in very wet years, water stays underground, surfacing farther to the east rather than here, but the footbridge remains. Hop on or walk alongside it to enter Pond Trail, which is where the loop begins.

Continue northwest through the shady oaks, cottonwood, and sycamores. You'll pass the exit marker for Upper Meadow Trail on the left. Keep going. About 0.25 miles in, you'll see a portable, chemical toilet restroom. A picnic table nearby on the north side of the trail in a small outlet overlooks the riverbed to the north. Stop and listen to the birds in this enchanted place, which was the first preserve owned by San Diego County. Saved from condominium builders in the 1970s, the land represents the county's first attempt to preserve a natural habitat and wilderness. Park rangers, along with the statewide organization Small Wilderness Area Preserves (SWAP), have worked hard to maintain the atmosphere that Ranger Judy Good calls "magical." Continue west toward the pond on this quiet, woodsy trail where poison ivy grows beneath the trees. Posted regulations encourage speaking softly, and forbid pets, loud music, or barbecues to protect the preserve's natural serenity.

A short distance ahead, a southward bend passes the ranger residence. The trail then heads west again, passing a kiosk with maps and information about ticks, which are common here. There is another chemical toilet to the south of the trail. A picnic table overlooks the man-made pond. The water level is kept low. In the 1950s this property was owned by Manchester Boddy, who intended to cultivate a botanical garden. He built the pond as part of a recirculating system to irrigate the camellias he planted. Take the short offshoot that leads around to the north edge of the pond for a closer look at the water. Here, the breeze causes the cattails to rustle softly and stirs up ripples in the sun-glinted water. The rapid music of the elusive wrentit and the low, vibrating sound of frogs fill the air. In summer, the cattails bloom in long, compact clusters that later open, releasing fluffy seeds that the wind blows around like cottony snow. Enjoy the peace before heading back to the main trail.

Head northwest where the trees grow thicker, pass by the Camellia View Trail exit marker, and, a little farther, that same trail's entrance. You're likely to see signs of wildlife here along the last 0.25 miles of the main trail. Raccoon and bobcat tracks, perhaps enlarged by gentle rains or nighttime moisture to look like bear or cougar tracks, mark the same trail you tread. Coyotes, deer, possum, and foxes also live here, but their natural shyness makes spotting them a rare occurrence. You're likely to see their droppings, though, and perhaps even get a whiff of skunk scent lingering somewhere along the path.

The trail halts at the end of the forest. Turn around and head southwest back to the Camellia View Trail entrance, now on your right. Enter the trail and head south. My family calls this area the "Tarzan" trail. Old-growth grapevines twist up through the trees. The deciduous vines turn to weathered, knotty ropes stretching up through oak branches in the winter, so no matter what the season, this section looks like a jungle. A rustic bench where the trail curves east provides a resting spot. Just be careful of poison oak amid the tangled foliage. In spring, the camellias bloom all around. In summer, clusters of grapes hang from the vines. The fruit is especially abundant in wetter years. Continuing along the trail, you'll cross a two-foot concrete spillway and then a wooden footbridge over a larger spillway. They were part of the irrigation system designed by Boddy but are now dry. Exit the 0.75-mile Camellia View Trail back near the pond and take the main trail south several yards to the entrance for the Upper Meadow Trail.

The Upper Meadow Trail heads southeast, gradually ascending through the trees along a river rock–lined path. You'll see holly-leaf cherry, toyon, and large boulders covered with sea foam–green lichen. The trail narrows, crosses a split-log bridge over a ravine, then becomes steeper as it briefly heads north. Curving east again, the trail opens up to meadows on the south side, then begins to descend. A set of steps made from railroad ties aids you in the steepest section. The ridge path overlooks the pond and the forested area below. Ferns cascade from the steep hillside wall like waterfalls, and moss covers sections of trail, tree trunks, and boulders. You'll hear the wrentit and woodpeckers, and see birds flitting among the trees. The route descends to level ground, meanders through a rocky section, and makes its way back to the main trail. From the Upper Meadow Trail exit sign, go right and head back across the wooden footbridge to the parking lot.

■ MORE FUN

After experiencing the peace and tranquility of nature, perhaps some excitement is in order. At nearby Pala Casino, 5 miles west on CA 76, the shrill sounds of slot machines advertising jackpot winnings will provide a contrast. Even if you don't gamble, Pala has six restaurants that offer everything from Asian food to steaks. The Terrace Room features an exhibition kitchen with 12 chefs preparing more than 60 food items. For more information, see **www.palacasino.com.**

■ TO THE TRAILHEAD

Take I-15 North past Escondido. Turn right on CA 76 East and drive about 10 miles, then turn right into the preserve.